RABIES
THE FACTS YOU NEED TO KNOW

G. N. HENDERSON
and KAY WHITE

First published in 1978 by
Barrie and Jenkins Ltd.,
24 Highbury Crescent, London N5 1RX

ISBN 0 214 20500 2

Typeset in Ehrhardt 'Monotype' by Jetset Typesetters, Brighton, Sussex

Printed in Great Britain by
William Clowes & Sons Limited, London, Beccles and Colchester

CONTENTS

Foreword

Having held responsibility for Britain's defences against rabies since October 1974, when the present legislation was still going through Parliament, and having introduced the present Rabies Awareness Campaign, it gives me considerable satisfaction to provide the foreword to this book.

The British government has made tremendous efforts to publicise our anti-rabies controls, and the reasons for them, both to the public at home and to potential visitors from overseas; indeed I believe that more effort has been put into publicity abroad for our import and quarantine regulations than has been done for any other piece of legislation. We are determined to remain free of rabies in this country, but to do so requires the cooperation and vigilance of us all. I view public awareness of the threat as a major weapon in our armoury.

Nevertheless it is very difficult for the government or a Ministry to describe in great detail either the threat itself or the countermeasures for dealing with it and to do so in an interesting and readable way. I believe that G. N. Henderson and Kay White have done a great service by filling this gap in a most comprehensive, responsible and realistic manner, while producing at the same time a book which is interesting and easily understandable to the average reader. It is not a veterinary textbook, but would not be out of place on any veterinary practitioner's bookshelf; at the same time it contains elements of history, drama and detection which could provide the plots for several films and novels.

The chapter dealing with an imaginary outbreak of the disease not only illustrates the way in which rabies could most easily be brought to Britain through selfishness or irresponsibility on the part of one individual, but describes the very comprehensive measures which would be used to control and eliminate the disease should an outbreak occur. These measures have been the subject of most careful and detailed planning by the authorities at both national and local level.

In preparing this book the authors have been in close consultation with

Ministry officials and veterinary officers. I am most grateful to them for their successful efforts to ensure a high degree of accuracy and, indeed, to take into account the most recent developments in policy, legislation and contingency planning. I commend their work to anyone who wishes to learn about or to improve his knowledge of rabies, and this should certainly include all those with an interest in or love for animals, whether as pets or as part of our wildlife heritage. We must know our enemy and rabies is a deadly enemy to us all.

Gavin Strang
Parliamentary Secretary
Ministry of Agriculture, Fisheries and Food

Introduction

The seas around Britain have been our defence against many enemies, not the least deadly of them being the dreaded rabies virus which destroys the brain of its victims, both human and animal, and inflicts terrible suffering before death as well as enormous strain and mental agony due to the very long incubation time before symptoms are manifest. Many countries live with rabies as part of their lives, but they also, however well they conceal it, live with fear. We in Britain put enormous value on our freedom to enjoy our countryside, to let our dogs run freely ahead of us unmuzzled, to pat a horse leaning over a gate or a cat sitting on a wall without any reservation that the friendly animal may do us irreparable harm or at best cause us weeks and months of nagging worry, because the strange animal might be rabid.

If rabies became established in Britain, as it is nearly all over Europe and in the Americas, the easy companionship we have with animals would end. People would still continue to keep pets, but there would be restraint and reservations; something very important to us would be lost, probably for ever.

The British Government is quite determined to keep rabies out of Britain and there is no reason why this should not be possible for it is a million to one chance that a rabid animal could get to this country . . . unless it is helped by a foolish, ignorant, or wicked person who smuggles in an animal without putting it through our protective quarantine barrier. By explaining what the rabies virus is, what it does, how it is transmitted, how we have kept it at bay for so long, this book seeks to reinforce the rabies awareness campaign mounted by the Ministry of Agriculture, Fisheries and Food, and supported so effectively by the veterinary profession, the local government authorities, the police, the National Health Service and many, many devoted dog and cat owners as well as those with sporting interests in animals.

The authors would like particularly to thank Mr Mick Loxam, CVO and Mr John Mcdonald, DVO of the Animal Health Division of MAFF at Tolworth, Surrey and Mr Jim Threlkeld, RVO at MAFF, Reading, for their invaluable help, Mrs Caroline O'Hagan for her work on the history of rabies, and the many members of the Royal College of Veterinary Surgeons who have cheerfully responded to requests for information and explanation. Freedom from rabies is a freedom very precious to us all, and it is a freedom that every person can help protect, by making sure that overseas visitors are aware of our regulations, but also by reporting those who appear to have broken them. By working together to this end, we can surely keep rabies out.

Kay White	G. N. Henderson, B.Sc., MRCVS
West Sussex	London

Chapter 1

Rabies: What It Is

Rabies, hydrophobia or lyssa are all names for the same dreaded disease, a long established scourge which we have no hope of eradicating in the foreseeable future. Only a handful of island countries are free of rabies, protected by the natural barrier of the sea. This geographical advantage, and our strict quarantine regulations which have been so wisely maintained in the face of considerable opposition in the past, has kept Britain free of any real outbreak of rabies for 50 years, but it is said that the disease waxes and wanes in one hundred year cycles, and we are now on the upturn to another rabies peak.

The very names by which the disease is known strike terror. Rabies is from the Latin word *rabere*, to rave, indicating the deranged mental state of the patient; hydrophobia, the fear of water which is one of the major signs of the disease in humans, and *lyssa*, the Greek word for frenzy, denoting the manic convulsions of brain fever induced by the virus. Rabies is essentially a virus disease of animals, which is transferred to man and other animals by means of a bite, or a lick on a sore place, or through the mucous membranes of mouth and eyes, or in the case of transference from the vampire bat, by breathing in virus particles from the air where bats have been present in great concentration, for example in caves or barns. Any warm-blooded animal, from a mouse or an elephant to a man may contract rabies, but some species, those which are normally "biters" are more prone to pass the disease on. There are, for instance, no recorded cases of rabies being passed from man to man in the past century, although modern intensive nursing techniques bring hospital staff in closer contact with the patient, so full protective measures are taken by those caring for the patient. The name "hydrophobia" is given only to the disease in humans, not to the disease in animals.

The rabies virus is classified as one of the Rhabdovirus group, the name taken from the Greek term for rod shaped. In the same group are found viruses which cause potato leaf curl, and a disease of the tobacco plant. The rabies virus is too small to be seen under an ordinary microscope but under the greater magnification of an electron microscope, the virus appears to be hood, or thimble shaped, with the outside surface covered in projecting spines. When the external covering is broken, a ribbon-like internal packing is released, containing ribonucleic acid, a substance found in the normal cells of the body, and having to do with cell reproduction. The rabies virus lives only in the nerve tissue and saliva of infected subjects. It has an incubation period of enormously variable time, from as little as 10 days to over a year, before a rapid upsurge in multiplication of the virus produces unendurable physical and mental symptoms which terminate in death of the victim once the stage of showing brain inflammation is reached. In recent months, claims have been made for the survival of two human patients with rabies infection confirmed, but one of these has severe brain damage.

Viruses invade the tissue cells of their host, by different routes according to the type of virus. Influenza virus is transmitted by droplet inhaled through the nose, poliomyelitis through the walls of the digestive system. All viruses destroy the cells of the body which they invade, and rabies characteristically destroys brain tissue. The majority of virus diseases do not respond to antibiotics and the sulpha-drugs which kill bacteria, but many virus diseases are being conquered by the use of vaccines and therein lies our defence, both of man and animals, in the face of rabies infection.

We can say with confidence that Britain is clear of rabies now, because as far as we are aware, no creature outside of quarantine kennels has the possibility of incubating the virus, and this state will remain, while there is no rabid animal in the country. Rabies is extremely unlikely to be contracted from any inanimate object like packaging, clothing or plant material. It will come in to this country, if it comes at all, by means of an animal which is incubating the disease; an animal which has not gone through our quarantine system spending six months in isolation.

Although the incubation for rabies is so long, the infected animal is not able to pass on the disease for the whole of the time. The virus only passes into the saliva of man or animal at the end of the incubation period, just before the warning symptoms are shown and after they are established, for the last few days of life. Getting an early warning of rabies behaviour is particularly difficult in the wild animal, where tell-tale changes in behaviour are not likely to be obvious. It is for this reason that the Ministry of Agriculture, Fisheries and Food (MAFF), have established the principle that an animal suspected of rabies must be retained in close confinement for 15 days, and if it is alive and well after that time, it could not have transmitted the disease (although it may still be incubating it). World Health Organisation information suggests that a 10 day interval is sufficient, but Britain's extra timing is in the interest of utmost safety.

Rabies has a most unusual disease pattern, quite different from the more familiar viral disease like measles, polio and mumps. With these infections the virus spreads via the bloodstream to the lymph glands where the virus multiplies, spreading to the target organ of the particular disease, the skin in measles, the spinal cord in polio, and the parotid gland, below and in front of the ear, in mumps. In all these diseases, the defence mechanisms of the body go into action at once, to prevent multiplication of the virus and in the end to destroy it and clear it out of the body. In a healthy person, after a period of misery, there will be recovery from the more common viral diseases, without any medication at all. It is only in rare cases, the very young, very old or very weak patient, where so many cells are destroyed that death takes place before the natural defence mechanism can eliminate the virus. Protection by vaccination which stimulates the system to produce its own antibodies to the disease is comparatively easy to establish against viral disease like smallpox and polio, and with so many of the world's population protected, these diseases are not the great threat they once were.

Rabies develops in quite a different way. It has an extremely long incubation period, which varies from case to case, followed by a progressive inflammation and breaking down of the central nervous system, when the disease spreads via the nerve cells to become concentrated in the area of the brain known as Ammon's Horn, where it destroys the cells it infects. This area of the brain, which runs across the middle of the head, from side to side, controls sensations of the tongue, face and neck, and movements of the legs, body and arms as well as speech. When a sufficient number of the brain cells have been destroyed so that the patient's use of the brain's functions is hampered, the obvious signs and symptoms of rabies occur. The virus spreads along the nerves in the outer parts of the body to reach other organs, particularly the salivary glands, the source of infection in a bite wound. Where brain cells are destroyed small black, oval or round clots are formed, known as Negri bodies. Negri was an Italian doctor who lived from 1876–1912, working at the University of Pavia in Italy at a time when it seemed that rabies would be conquered, following the work of Louis Pasteur. Negri's discovery of these black bodies in the brain cells of rabies victims resulted in the establishment of the search for Negri bodies at postmortem becoming one of the standard tests for rabies for many years. Once the brain cells have been invaded by rabies, and destruction of cells has begun, the progress of the disease cannot be stopped even with the most sophisticated medical knowledge which we have at our disposal today, mainly because the body itself puts up such a poor defence. One advantage we have against rabies is that the long incubation period allows steps to be taken to prevent the disease developing *after* a person has been exposed to rabies. This is not possible in the more common viral diseases like influenza and measles. Provided medical help is sought at once, after a bite or a lick from a suspected animal in a country where there is rabies, anti-rabies vaccine can be given to stimulate production of antibodies before the virus starts to multiply and move from the site of the bite into the nervous system.

Rabies virus is easily killed by sunlight, heat, formalin and standard disinfectants; after thorough cleaning, there need be no fear that the virus will linger on the premises where a rabid animal has been. The virus dies in dried saliva within a few hours, but it may be shed in urine, faeces and milk, and persist in the carcase of a dead animal for about 24 hours, depending on climatic conditions. Gamebirds, pheasant and partridge which have been savaged by a rabid fox could be dangerous to handle.

Every time the waves of rabies infection reach their peak, changes in economic conditions and situations result in different animals being the most frequently affected. Early in this century, rabies was a disease of dogs, but now the dog is quite low on the list of susceptible animals. In France now, foxes are by far the most commonly affected animals with farm animals next and then cats and dogs. In America, the order goes . . . skunks, foxes, bats, raccoons, with dogs next and then cats. In relation to the total number of cases, dogs come very low on both lists. In India the large population of stray and semi-wild dogs act as constant reservoirs of infection, so there is no possibility of the country becoming clear of the disease.

The susceptibility of the different species and the symptoms which they present vary a great deal, and in the individual, they vary again. All animals may be affected by either one, or both, or a mixture of the two recognised forms of rabies, the Furious or frenzied form, and Dumb Rabies, when violent symptoms are absent and a gradual creeping paralysis precedes a quiet death. Neither of these forms are absolutely clear cut and there may be episodes of each type of behaviour in either form. In general, it is said that the meat eating animals, including man, are more likely to show the furious form, biting and raving uncontrollably, but they may also fade into coma before reaching the maniac stage. Cattle, sheep and goats are never very efficient biters, and in rabies they are likely to become paralysed in the jaw muscles at an early stage, so they are not so likely to inflict bites, and to pass on the virus.

The course of rabies in the fox, badger, squirrel, rat and rabbit is similar to that seen in the dog. Following the bite of a rabid animal, signs are likely to be seen in from two to eight weeks, or longer, the incubation varying with the amount of virus transmitted, the size of the bite and where it was located on the body. A deep bite on mouth or face being of more significance to the speed with which virus is transmitted to the brain than a slight wound on the foot which may take six months to produce symptoms or may never do so at all. Analysis of rabies cases in dogs within quarantine premises in this country show that half occurred within one month of importation and nearly all within four months. The animals may have been infected at varying intervals before they were brought to Britain, but our quarantine period of six months is therefore quite adequate.

Chapter 2

The History of Rabies

There are many references to what is almost certainly rabies in the recorded history of several civilisations, and, as we learn more about the disease from both the past and the present, we find it almost as fascinating as it is unpleasant. It is remarkable to note that basic behaviour of rabies virus was well understood by the Babylonian law-makers of 2300 BC. They imposed a fine on the owner of any rabid dog who failed to confine it so as to prevent it attacking anyone, although admittedly modern man might not approve the lower fine levied if the bitten person was a slave.

A Greek writer called Democritus described rabies in his chronicles between five and four hundred years before the time of Christ, as did Aristotle in about 322 BC. Strangely, the latter, whose observations were often so acute, only recognised rabies as a disease of animals. It was Celsus who wrote of the transmissibility between species. An illness that can be passed from any other species to man is called a zoonose, and is of great interest to physicians and veterinarians. One year after the birth of Christ, a doctor hit on the idea of cauterising a bitewound inflicted by a rabid animal with liquids, and he would no doubt be gratified to hear that the WHO officially recommended similar techniques in 1966. For many years and in several lands it was thought advisable to immerse people exposed to rabies repeatedly in the sea; the benefits of this are dubious, but weak salt solution applied immediately after the infliction of a skin injury and for a few days afterwards is good first aid procedure.

Among the writings of Robert Burton in the 17th century, transmission of rabies from dog to man is discussed, and about 150 years later the Englishman Jesse Foot remarked that, in his experience, not all those bitten by rabid dogs became ill with rabies. It was, in fact, very hard for the doctors in his day to be sure when a dog really had the disease, because distemper, epilepsy, brain tumours and head injury could all cause similar signs, and there were no "path. labs" to send samples to. Foot encouraged amputation of the bitten part, which was a sound idea in theory, but had the disadvantage that less than half the victims survived the ordeal in dirty surroundings and without the benefit of anaesthesia.

The first one hears of efficient rabies control by dog-owners is in 1794, when a British master of foxhounds imposed a quarantine or isolation period on all new stock introduced into his kennels – a policy still in use in many island states today. Bardsley, a doctor of medicine, had the foresight to recommend a national quarantine and the prohibiton of import of dogs to Britain in 1807, but his idea was rejected, the disease not being alarmingly common at the time, while dog-fanciers needed to buy new strains from abroad. French legal records of 1821 describe how a judge awarded 8,000 francs to a widow against the owner of a rabid dog which had bitten her husband, apparently causing his death. The child of an English labourer subsequently had the ill luck to be bitten by the tethered rabid dog of an innkeeper. The child died, and his father claimed the surgeon's and the undertaker's fees, but the innkeeper was ordered to pay the larger sum of £36 in court.

In 1828 a surgeon called Sully realised that the advantages of excising (cutting out) tissues contaminated by the bite or saliva of a rabid animal were partly offset by the danger of carrying rabies particles on the surgeon's scalpel to the rest of the patient's body, which represented something of a breakthrough in operating theatre technique. It is easy for us to understand how disease organisms behave when we can see photographs or even cine film of them, but at the time of Sully many so-called dog experts genuinely believed rabies was the result of poor food and kennel management. Even some people who understood how rabies could be passed on from dogs to other animals thought it arose "spontaneously" in the canine race – rather as it had been supposed at one stage that baby mice were not borne by female mice, but arose magically out of rubbish heaps.

Four thousand years of rabies history may be dismissed thus in a few sentences, but they help to set the stage for Louis Pasteur, Antoni van Leeuwenhoek, Robert Koch and some of the other geniuses whose major discoveries enabled medicine to begin to crack the problem of this excruciating illness.

Look first at the study of infectious disease and of microscopy. Before disease organisms were made visible to the human eye by lens systems, the concept of a "living contagium" gained and lost favour amongst medical men from time to time. It was appreciated that some diseases could spread amongst people sharing a common environment, rather as mould might spread through a bowl of oranges. Then van Leeuwenhoek, born in 1632, found that by arranging lenses in a complicated system he could achieve enormous magnifications – and that, provided he illuminated his subjects brightly enough, he could see in detail things that were invisible to the naked eye. The much-quoted remark about the microscope revealing a whole world of which mankind was previously ignorant is not in the least extravagant. Novelists would have been proud to have dreamed up the world which van Leeuwenhoek and his followers actually realised. It was Pasteur and Koch who used his invention to get closer to the minute living creatures that fascinated them, and so lay the foundations of what we call bacteriology. Pasteur's life has been well documented.

He was born in Burgundy in 1822, and attended the Ecole Normale in Paris. On completion of his schooling, he became assistant to his ex-teacher, who luckily allowed him to do some original work. Pasteur discovered by a series of chemical experiments why tartaric and para-tartaric (sometimes called racemic) acids behaved differently from one another, although it was impossible to tell them apart analytically. Later, other chemists, repeating his experiments with other substances, found that a certain class of chemicals obeys certain rules – and the members are still known today as stereochemicals. Perhaps some of the credit for Pasteur's expertise should go to Claude Bernard, who wrote a textbook on experimental method, and whom young Louis greatly admired.

On leaving Paris, he went to teach at Dijon and Strasbourg, and later he was appointed Dean of the Faculty of Natural Science at Lille. The local major industry was the production of alcohol (for human consumption), and so Pasteur made fermentation his main study-project. At one point he was working on beer with a colleague who enjoyed the sampling of their research-product infinitely more than Pasteur. At last they produced in the lab what they had been aiming for. The colleague took a mouthful of the brew and beamed: "It's perfect", he announced. Pasteur had a sip, spat it out and fetched a microscope. A few moments later, still scowling with distaste, he concurred. It was fortunate that Pasteur studied alcoholic fermentation first, because the "causal organism" is a yeast – a comparatively large microbe. He went on to discover that the souring of milk, the rancidification of butter and the deterioration of wine into vinegar are all caused by microbes that are even smaller, and which we call anaerobic bacteria – members of the one-celled plant group that flourish in conditions where there is no oxygen. He also found out that heat kills these anaerobes, this process being quickly put to practical use in the wine industry, whose grateful organisers called it "pastuerisation". The English always think of this in connection with milk, but the French have their gastronomic priorities right. The study of anaerobes was in dispute until Pasteur had exploded the myth of "spontaneous generation", proving that microbes actually reproduce themselves, rather than materialising out of thin air, and this was finally accepted by the scientific world. By this time he had inspired a considerable amount of faith in his own country, and was consulted on a number of topics. One of these was an outbreak of the disease Pebrine among silkworms in Southern France, where silk producers became worried about the drastically lowered output and the rapid spread from farm to farm. The great chemist had a harder task this time, as the causal organism was a virus and too small to be seen under the microscopes available in 1865, but he still managed to propose control methods which worked.

He next studied two bacillary diseases (diseases caused by the bacteria called bacillae) of farm animals – chicken cholera and splenic fever, which affects sheep, cattle and also Man (nowadays called Anthrax). People who had experimented with chickens infected with chicken cholera in the past had found that they could reproduce the disease in healthy birds if they injected them with tissues taken from the sick birds and mixed up with fluid. Pasteur did roughly the same, but using infected material that had been kept for a while. This caused a milder form of the disease in the previously fit birds, with no fatalities. What was more, if these experimental chickens came into contact with cholera-infected ones much later, they stayed uninfected – they were immune. It would be grossly unfair to overlook the work of Jenner, who in 1798 had used cowpox material to protect humans against a related disease, smallpox; but Pasteur's achievements with chicken cholera are important in the history of immunisation because he was the first to render a disease organism less harmful – a process known to this day as attenuation. He continued the useful work by supervising the mass-production of vaccines for use against chicken cholera, swine fever and Anthrax. Thus armed with experience and to some extent boosted by the confidence shown in him by men of public standing, Louis Pasteur began to tackle the villain of this book – rabies.

The science of immunology was a comparatively new one, but the practice of immunology was very old, rather as primitive Man had learned to build seaworthy boats long before Archimedes' Principle explained why it was they stayed afloat. Nowadays we like to understand why things work, and the fact that such remedies as faith-healing, homeopathy and acupuncture sometimes succeed where scientific medicine fails may lead to scepticism. For centuries, however, people were encouraged by such authorities as the Christian priesthood to regard illness and recovery as events beyond the control of Man.

One early reference to the use of preventive medicine is the mention of Mithridates, King of Pontus, who was apparently frightened of being poisoned by his enemies. He fed various poisons in low dosages to some ducks, which he then killed in order to drink their blood. The next lot of ducks got slightly higher dosages, and so the king developed a tolerance to the poisons – not quite the same as an immunity to bacterial or viral disease, but effected by the same principle. Later, Pliny the Elder, whose diaries were luckily preserved for posterity, wrote that he thought that it would be a good idea to eat the livers of dogs that had died of rabies if you wanted to avoid developing the disease. This may sound quite repulsive, but many modern vaccines are prepared from infected animal tissue, purified, and then administered on sugar-lumps.

In the East, it was discovered in early times that the discharge taken from the vesicles (blisters) of patients suffering from mild bouts of smallpox could be introduced by scratching into the skin of healthy subjects, who then became immune. In 1721, Lady Mary Wortley Montagu, whose husband had been in the diplomatic service in Turkey, introduced the technique into Britain. By 1798, Jenner found that immunity to smallpox could be effected by the use of cowpox material. This is because the smallpox organism is a cousin of the cowpox one, and the body's immune mechanism cannot distinguish between the two, but releases the same combatting fluids and corpuscles to deal with them. A further invention necessary for the progress of immunology was made by the Edinburgh University lecturer, Alexander Wood, for to him we owe the hypodermic syringe.

Meanwhile, studies of the biology of immunity had produced two schools of thought; Pasteur's pupil, Metchnikoff, thought phagocytosis protected us from disease, while the Cambridge man, Nuttall, demonstrated in the lab that the body forms fluids containing antibodies. Phagocytosis is a word of Greek origin – "Phago" meaning eating, "cyte" a cell, and "-osis" the process of. In other words, the process of cells eating, and they "eat" the disease organisms. We now know that it is necessary for the antibodies Nuttall discovered to knock out these organisms before the phagocytes can eat them. But the interesting part is that, while the phagocytes obligingly eat up any dead bodies they come across, the antibodies are specific – that is to say there is one type that combats measles, another whooping cough, another mumps, and so on; and once the body has been educated to produce, say, measles antibody, it never forgets how. The discovery of the specificity of antibodies may actually be accredited to a pupil of Koch's called Pfeiffer, who showed in the lab that the organism *cholera vibrios* was neutralised by antibodies made by an immunised guinea pig.

There was yet another discovery to be made, and Pasteur's associate, Pierre Roux, made it, in 1888. In some diseases, it is not the organism that makes the patient sick, but a substance called a toxin, which it exudes. If you can produce some of this toxin in the lab, you can use it like a vaccine. Diphtheria and tetanus are two illnesses in which antitoxins are used. Another famous biologist, Ehrlich, explained the difference between passive and active immunity in 1892. Both sorts are needed in the treatment of rabies.

Contemporary with Louis Pasteur were Jenner, whose bold trials in the use of a vaccine against smallpox in man were successful, and Toussaint, who discovered that liquid preparations of disease organisms lost some of their power to produce illness if they were heated or treated with carbolic acid (phenol). The famous English surgeon, Lister, was later to use this same substance to kill the germs in his operating theatre, thus greatly reducing the number of fatalities from post-operative infection.

Pasteur's study of the prophylaxis (preventive treatment) of rabies began in 1880 and continued for about five years. Possibly he selected this disease because of memories of a rabid wolf that attacked men and animals in the district of Jura in his early childhood, causing the death of eight people. The fact that he was 59 and crippled by a stroke when he began the research is some indication of his courageous spirit. He was assisted in he project by Roux, a medical man, and Chamberland, a bacteriological technician, inventor of the autoclave and the bacterial filter, both of which have been used widely in medicine for over a century. Working on rabbits infected with rabies, Pasteur found that, when the disease was transmitted to a series of individuals, it eventually reached a stage where the incubation period became fixed at six days. Samples of the virus showing this behaviour he named "fixed virus", to distinguish it from the naturally-occurring virus, which he named "street virus". Oddly enough, the potency of the virus did not show consistency, fixed virus obtained from rabbits causing rabies in a higher percentage of dogs than fixed virus obtained from monkeys. It became clear that here was a dangerous and unpredictable customer! Next Pasteur's team tried to weaken the virus by drying samples of spinal cords of rabies-infected rabbits. They felt that if the organism could be weakened (or attenuated, as it is now called), it might be suitable for injection into patients in order to stimulate the production of anti-rabies antibodies. Several years of work on dogs revealed that they could develop immunity against rabies by a progressively potent series of injections; first day, dog injected with rabbit spinal cord that had been dried for 14 days; second day, dog injected with rabbit spinal cord that had been dried for 13 days; and so on for 15 days. Why drying reduced the potency of rabies in the spinal cords is still not understood. Perhaps it reduced the numbers of live organisms.

Word got out that Pasteur's team was having some success, and in 1885 poor little Joseph Meister, aged nine, was brought from Alsace, in the hope that he could be saved. He had been bitten no less than 14 times by a rabid dog on the hands and legs. His doctor thought he was already doomed to die, and that Pasteur's vaccine certainly could not make him worse and might possibly make him better. Faced with the prospect of using his crude product on a child, Pasteur was conscience-stricken, while Rous divorced himself from the project altogether. The child's physician, however, took responsibility. Sixty hours after the bites occurred, Joseph was given a shot of spinal cord that had been dried for a fortnight. The next day he received 13-days-dried cord, and so on for a total of 12 daily doses. He then returned to Alsace, and to everyone's delight and amazement, survived. When he grew up, Joseph returned to become the porter at the Institute Pasteur. He finally came to a tragic end when he committed suicide rather than admit troops of the German army to Pasteur's burial chamber in 1940.

At the end of the year 1885, the 14-year-old shepherd Jean-Baptiste Jupille came to Pasteur. He had been bitten defending some younger boys from a rabid dog (which he finally succeeded in killing, a difficult task for one not carrying weapons). Treatment began six days after the bites were sustained, and the injections followed the same pattern as those given to Joseph Meister. Jupille survived. Present day knowledge of rabies suggests that, since treatment was initiated late, Jupille would possibly not have developed rabies even if he had gone without treatment, for statistics show that a certain percentage of people bitten by animals later proved to be rabid survive although they receive no vaccine. At the time of Jupille's salvation, however, the scientific and medical worlds were inclined to attribute success to Pasteur, and there can be little doubt that, from a moral point of view, he earned it.

Soon after this triumph, a girl called Louise Pelletier was brought to Pasteur 37 days after being bitten on the face. Any modern doctor would view such a case with the utmost gloom, and it is hardly surprising that the patient died 11 days after the end of Pasteur's treatment. His detractors at once claimed this death as proof of the vaccine's inefficacy, and destructive criticisms of Pasteur and his team continued, although his success rate with 2,500 patients over the following 15 months, far exceeded his failure rate.

In 1887 Pasteur suffered further strokes, resulting in temporary loss of speech.

The 2,500 rabies patients who reached Pasteur in the years 1885–1887 have been mentioned as a mere statistic. A close observation of one of the victims would be helpful.

> Alexey's wrists and ankles, which had been chafed at the beginning of the journey, were now reduced to a bleeding, smarting mess by the coarse rope that bound him to his iron bedstead. As the train pounded on across monotonous steppes, he would catch occasional glimpses of dripping icicles, streams swollen with melt-water, or flooded fields. At this, his Adam's apple would bob involuntarily as his gorge rose in disgust, and his eyes, already wild, would dilate

still further in uncomprehending terror, while the bound arms tried helplessly to ward off the dreaded water. Darkness brought him some respite, but the sound of his attendant approaching soon filled him with a fresh agony of apprehension. The grim-faced man entered the compartment with caution, glanced at his patient with a mixture of revulsion and pity, and left. A draught of cold air brushed Alexey's throat as he did so, causing it to convulse as it did whenever he saw water. His brain was in a turmoil; the feelings of thirst that tormented him after two days without water battling against the instincts that prevented him from allowing it to pass his lips. His body twitched at intervals and there was no rest other than periods a few seconds long when he tucked his head into his chest in a gesture of withdrawal and remained motionless. He could understand nothing, and perhaps it was this ignorance that made his fear so acute.

After an indeterminable time, in which daylight brought real water, and darkness watery nightmares, the train stopped. Three new attendants stepped into the compartment and, avoiding Alexey's gaze and keeping as far as possible from his head, manoeuvred the bed on to a farm cart that had been drawn alongside. It had a cover of canvas, but was open back and front. At a word from the attendants, the driver shrugged as though to rid himself of the monster in his vehicle, and drove rapidly away. Pasteur's hospital and research establishment were eight hours' drive from the railway station, and these eight hours would be re-lived often in the dreams and stories of the cart driver.

This ugly story is a fictitious account of a real journey, but the records indicate that the treatment and sensations of the rabies victim are authentic. When Louis Pasteur was investigating the course of the disease, he needed rabies cases to study and to try out his vaccines upon, and some of these were supplied by the current Tsar of Russia and shipped, with suitable restraint, by rail to the Institut. It appears that the majority of these were peasants bitten by wolves affected by a rabies enzootic. From their point of view a sudden, forcible rail journey to France would have been bewildering even if they had been mentally normal at the time; and the treatment did not always benefit them when they arrived in any event. But from a detached point of view, we may conclude that Pasteur was sufficiently well-regarded for influential people to help him in his work, and sufficiently single-minded to work repeatedly with very distressing cases. Furthermore, his research, while not resulting in a perfect rabies cure in his lifetime, opened up a whole new school of thought on both vaccines and rabies.

Chapter 3

Rabies in 19th Century Britain

As long as rabies has been known in the world, people have been looking for a "cure" for it, even now unsuccessfully, as will be shown in the stories of the three rabies victims who died in Britain during 1976. There was for a long time a strong belief that the first puppy from the first litter of a bitch would never become rabid, but it is not possible to discover any basis for this belief. The variability of the presence of virus in the saliva of even an obviously rabid animal must have given rise to the idea that some people and animals even when bitten were mysteriously protected from taking the disease.

North American Indians believed that the names Melampo, Cubilon, and Lubina would protect dogs against rabies, for these were the names of the dogs which followed the shepherds to Bethlehem to gaze upon the face of the infant Christ. Several saints in the Catholic hierarchy are said to possess the power to protect against rabies: St Dominic of Tuscany, who lived in AD 304, Parthenius, a fourth century bishop of Asia Minor, and St Ulric, who cured rabies by the touch of his cross are most frequently mentioned. St Hubert is the special protector of dogs. On his patronal day, November 2nd, little cakes blessed on his altar would be fed to dogs to keep them safe from rabies for a year, and pilgrimages were made to his shrine for rabies cures. St Vitus was also a patron saint of dogs, invoked against dog bites and "all hurts that dogs can do to men". St Roche, who lived from 1298 to 1327 in France also had a cake giving ceremony on his day, August 16th, when dogs were taken to his altar to be blessed and get their protective biscuit for the year. It is interesting that St Roche's day falls in high summer, during the dog days when dogs are supposed to be particularly prone to madness. There was also a longstanding theory that newborn dogs have a "worm" beneath the tongue, which if it is removed, deprives them of the power of biting should they become rabid. The "worm" was probably a small ligament beneath the tongue which had no effect at all on biting mechanism.

In *Chambers Information for the People* of 1842, a publication described as "scientific and general knowledge suitable for the wants of the middle and labouring classes" there is a fair description of the symptoms of rabies, but some uncertainty as to how the first case in any area can originate; there is no conception that a rabies reservoir may remain in wildlife. The most modern thought at that time was that human rabies was only a nervous affection, arising from the imagination – "the person fancies he is going mad, and mad he becomes". The authors thought it wise still to take every available precaution, and "on being bit, it is always safe to wash the wound immediately, and have the parts burnt with a hot iron, or cut out". The famous Hertfordshire cure, known as Webb's drink, was concocted as follows: "Take the fresh leaves of the tree box, two ounces; fresh leaves of rue, two ounces; of sage, half an ounce; chop these finely and boil in a pint of water until it reduces to half a pint. Strain and press out the liquor. Beat the leaves in a mortar to bruise thoroughly, and boil them again in a pint of new milk, press the leaves out as before. After this, mix both the boiled liquors, which will make three doses for a human subject. Double this quantity will make three doses for a horse or cow, two-thirds is sufficient for a large dog, calf or sheep or hog, half the quantity for a middle-sized dog and one-third for a smaller one." The doses were to be given first thing in the morning after an overnight fast, and three were said to be sufficient. A lecturer in chemistry had different ideas, culled from his own science. He advised, in a letter to a newspaper, "Let a mixture of two parts of nitric and one part of muriatic acid, both by measure, evolving chlorine in a concentrated form, be applied to the wound as soon as possible, and more than once".

In 1813, 14 rabies victims at a Moscow hospital were successfully treated by a peasant healer with a decoction of tops and blossoms of Genista, the broom plant, of which they had to consume 3 kilos each day. Twice daily the patients were examined for knots under the tongue, in which it was believed the virus would be found. When they appeared, the knots were opened and cauterised with a red hot wire, and the patients were said to have recovered in six weeks, while patients treated more conventionally by the physicians of the hospital died. It was thought that rabies became absorbed from the bite wound and for a short time remained beneath the tongue. If the tongue knots were not opened when they appeared, at the third to ninth day after the bite, the virus would be absorbed into the system and the patient would die. It is interesting to see how knowledge about rabies progressed, sometimes near to our present theories, and sometimes digressing – we know now that rabies does affect the salivary glands especially, but much later in the disease, after a long incubation.

At the time of the battle of Waterloo (1815), rabid dogs were a common sight on the streets of London; one running down Park Lane was said to have bitten five horses and as many dogs. The fashionable Dalmatian, running with the gentleman's carriage, was not infrequently bitten by a cur dog; the Dalmatian infected the horse by licking its muzzle, and then the coachman fell victim to the same infection: three deaths from the one bite. There was quite accurate observation of rabies symptoms, acute restlessness being the earliest to show and then severe pain in the ear, the most likely site of the bite. As much as five grains of opium would be administered to a dog in the violent phase in a vain effort to quieten its convulsions.

Diagnosis of dog rabies at this time lay either in opening up the stomach to see if the dog had been consuming excreta, sticks and stones in the depraved appetite syndrome common to the rabid dog, or in "procuring a poor worthless cur dog and getting him bitten by the suspect animal, and then to carry the disease to a third victim". It was realised that saliva could carry rabies virus as a footman died through handling a pet spaniel which had been rolled over and made dirty, but not bitten, by a rabid dog. Animal and human doctors marvelled at the variability of rabies virus; they knew that of four dogs bitten only three would show rabid symptoms and in humans, only one out of four would become rabid. They knew that the incubation time varied, maintaining that some would show rabid symptoms on the day they were bitten, while others did not become rabid until twelve or even thirty years after the original encounter, but four or five months was thought to be the average time, not far from our modern assessment.

Youatt, the unqualified doctor, knew that rabies virus must be received into a wound, but Professor Dick, founder of Edinburgh School of Veterinary Medicine, thought that rabies was an inflammation of the nose and an occasional epidemic similar to influenza. In the human, it was "merely the melancholy, a product of disordered imagination". Youatt felt that if *every dog in the country* could be separately confined for eight months the disease would be extinguished but realised that such a revolutionary idea would not be popular with the sporting world and not enforceable with the peasantry. His more rational proposal was that a tax should be laid on every useless dog, the cur and lurcher in the country, the fighting dog in the town . . . in this idea he was at least thirty years ahead of his time.

No attempt was made to treat rabid animals: for the human patient, the method was to widely open up the wound, cutting away all tissue where the animal tooth had touched, and then to pour on caustic made of caustic and nitric acid after cleaning the site with a stream of boiling water poured on from a kettle . . . and this at a time when inhaled anaesthetics had not been discovered! When the ensuing dead tissue was sloughed off, it was thought the virus was wrapped up in it and rendered harmless. The caustic treatment often had to be repeated if the wound was infected at the bottom, and the procedure was seldom effective. Small wonder that the parents of a child which had been bitten smothered it with pillows rather than see such suffering inflicted in vain.

In Vienna, in the year 1887, a law was passed by which, if a dog was rabid and bit a man, the dog's owner was liable to a year's imprisonment, the first time that the onus for protecting fellow men had been put on a dog's owner, and the first direct evidence that it was known that dogs could be protected from rabies other than by magic; if dogs were restricted in movement and kept under control, they would not become rabid. A muzzling order for all dogs except packs of hounds had been in existence for two years in an attempt to eradicate rabies from the city. There was a muzzling order in Britain too, but by 1896, rabies cases were becoming rarer in Britain and people were restive about having to muzzle their dogs. At a public meeting in protest, two prominent gentlemen, one a veterinary surgeon, declared their disbelief in rabies as a disease. People have always been very ready to believe that if they do not see rabies, it has gone away. There was still, 11 years after Louis Pasteur had successfully treated a boy bitten by a mad dog, doubts about the vaccine treatment. Although Pasteur himself had always said that his vaccine would be of no use if applied after symptoms had developed, people would insist on confusing the preventative treatment with a cure. It was said in Britain that the supporters of the Pasteur Institut could not point to a single case of positive cure. This of course was true, as all the successes had come with patients bitten but not yet showing the rabies symptoms. Several patients who came to Pasteur too late did succumb to the disease, and his detractors were quick to seize on his failures, some were inclined to say the whole treatment was a fraud and that Pasteur was a murderer, and that those who died were killed by the treatment rather than the disease. It is understandable that it was difficult for the ordinary person to grasp the idea of giving, if even in the mildest form, a deadly disease to someone who already had run the risk of contracting that disease. There still exists a faction of people, primarily those interested in nature cures and homoeopathic medicine, who are opposed to the idea of vaccination against infectious disease in man and animals, believing, as Dr Margery Blackie states in her book, *The Patient, not the Cure* – "infectious diseases themselves play a part in the development of a child and the naturally produced immunity is so much more valuable than that produced by injections . . . one of the values of having an infectious disease can be seen in the clearing up of eczema after an attack of measles". This theory may have substance when used about the virus diseases from which the body will recover, given good care, in any case, but rabies is not one of those diseases. During 1895 the Pasteur Institut in Paris treated 1,500 patients of which only five died, so there were good grounds for thinking that rabies might not be the death sentence it once was. The name Pasteur became a magical one for those threatened with the consequences of animal bites, and it was said that 19 Russian men, who had been savaged by a mad wolf, made the journey to Paris to seek his help, repeating the only French word they knew, "Pasteur, Pasteur". The name was a talisman which carried them to the saviour's door, but some were gravely ill when they arrived, having travelled overland for two weeks, but of the 19, 16 survived and went home again. The Tsar contributed 100,000 francs towards the building of the Pasteur Institut as an expression of gratitude. Many people from all over France subscribed also to building the fine laboratories and treatment rooms. Many countries established their own Pasteur Institutes, so that their countrymen did not have to make the lengthy journey to Paris; for some time Britain was the only major country where the treatment was not available, until the Institute of Preventative Medicine was opened in Chelsea, and the Pasteur system was applied there.

Treatment at the Pasteur Institut in Paris was entirely free, no fees were charged or would be accepted. Grateful patients and others became subscribers to the Institute if they wished, but this gave them no priority of treatment in case of need. There was no in-patient care, and no other medication other than the innoculation for which patients attended every morning for 15 days, spending the rest of the time as they wished. Many of the patients lodged at a hotel in the vicinity of the Institut in the Rue Edmund Guillot, said to be very comfortable and extraordinarily cheap, and where the proprietor understood all the requirements of the Institut and also spoke English fluently. As people were still very wary indeed of submitting to vaccination, another rabies treatment to gain favour was by means of steam baths, taken one or more times daily, in conjunction with Belladonna (deadly nightshade) pills by mouth, for six months at least. Belladonna is still used in homoeopathic medicine to reduce fever. If in spite of the medication, the rabies symptoms developed, the instructions were to place the patient in a Turkish bath and to keep him in it.

A patent recipe for the cure of hydrophobia was kept in most British households at the turn of the century. One reads: Hydrophobia may be prevented, by means of the following treatment. The first dose is 2 ounces of coltsfoot root, bruised, in one pint of new milk which has been reduced to one half by boiling. Take all at one dose in the morning, fasting till the afternoon. The second dose should be two ounces of coltsfoot in milk as before, and the third the same. Three doses are sufficient to remove all ill effects of the bite. A dose for a horse or cow should be four times the above. A treatment for dogs bitten by another with rabies was by the administration of eight to twelve grains of turpeth mineral mixed into a pill with conserve of roses. This pill to be given for three days together and repeated the night preceding the full moon and change of two or three successive moons. Turpeth mineral is made from the stem and root of the plant Ipomaea (Morning Glory), and is a purgative.

These home remedies stood at least a 50:50 chance of being "successful" owing to the variable nature of the infection, so some of the more lucky recipes probably acquired reputations as infallible cures.

In 1874 an outbreak of street rabies resulted in over 70 deaths among humans; by 1890 the government had made the wearing of muzzles by dogs compulsory in danger areas. Controls on the importation of dogs to

Great Britain were introduced by an order made in 1897 when a form of house quarantine was required and the incidence of rabies was very much reduced. In view of the present epidemic of wild life rabies both in Europe and in the Americas, it is surprising that there is no record that rabies has ever been widespread among foxes in the British countryside, but in 1886 there was an outbreak among the protected deer kept in Richmond Park.

Rabies was re-introduced into the country as a result of one or more pet dogs being smuggled in on a returning troop ship at the end of World War I. There were 319 rabies outbreaks, all but a few of the cases being in dogs. Muzzling orders were enforced and there were many prosecutions of those doting owners who would insist on taking their dogs out without the restricting muzzle. The most difficult dogs to fit with protective headgear were the Pekinese, very much in vogue as ladies' pets.

1928 brought legislation enforcing six months quarantine for imported dogs and cats, the quarantine period to be passed in approved kennels. From that time until October 1969 no case of rabies occurred outside quarantine premises and only 27 animals died of rabies while in quarantine. Several times during this forty years of safety a wave of protest was initiated by dog lovers. They wanted the quarantine time shortened or abolished, for it seemed that the danger and the threat of rabies had passed and new generations of dog lovers had forgotten the mortal fear. Those interested in exhibiting dogs at shows were, and still are, especially keen to have free exchange of dogs between Britain, USA and Europe for the purpose of stimulating competition and so that foreign dogs could be brought here to be used at stud, so enlarging the pool of hereditable genes.

Chapter 4

The Vaccines of the 20th Century

In order to understand the present-day methods of combating rabies, it is necessary to consider briefly some of the more important development in the field of immunology after Pasteur's work finished.

In 1888 Pasteur's associate Pierre Roux demonstrated that some disease organisms, of which diphtheria is an example, produce noxious substances called toxins, which are responsible for illness in the patient. This made possible the later manufacture and use of antitoxins in medicine.

In 1892 Ehrlich explained the processes of passive and active immunisation. This led, in time, to the ability of physicians to provide immediate treatment for patients exposed to infectious disease and or preventive treatment when it was possible to anticipate exposure.

Ernest Goodpasture discovered a way to avoid the use of live animals in the production of vaccines in 1933. He grew disease organisms on the membranes of chicken eggs, which were kept in an incubator. This method is still widely used at the present day, and accounts for the fact that people who are allergic to eggs may not be given certain vaccines.

Despite the efficacy of the vaccines made and used in the late 19th and early 20th centuries, a number of unpleasant side-effects were reported, and the technique of vaccination could easily have fallen into disrepute and been discarded, had it not been for the passing of the Therapeutic Substances Act in Great Britain in 1925, which ensured that only pure, safe and effective "biologicals" reached the market.

"Pasteur treatment" of exposed persons continued in Europe and the faith doctors grew to have in it is backed up by a report published in 1916, stating that 0.6% of treated patients died, as compared with 16% of untreated ones. All the victims in the report were definitely exposed to rabies, as proved by laboratory tests on the animals which bit them. It is interesting that these figures for mortality in bitten patients agree with those published in the 1970s.

Let us now look at the rabies situation in Europe in general, and Great

Britain in particular, for the period from 1887 to 1975.

Pasteur's work on the pre-exposure treatment of dogs was repeated soon after his retirement from active life. Several sources confirmed that it is possible to render dogs immune to rabies by giving them a course of injections of suitably-prepared rabies virus, and that humans may be similarly protected. What the experimenters did not elucidate – and this question is still unanswered today – was why the introduction of laboratory virus with a needle triggers the development of immunity, while the introduction of "street" virus with a tooth does not. What exactly have those rabbits, chickens' eggs or other live tissues done to weaken the virus, to disarm it, so that the body can tackle it successfully?

Institutes modelled on the Pasteur Institut in France sprang up all over the world. By 1889 there were 79 institutes in Russia; five in Italy; one in Vienna; one in Bucharest; one in Barcelona; one in Rio de Janeiro; one in Buenos Aires; one in Havana; and one in Mexico. The British Government chose however, to adopt an altogether different policy towards rabies. Instead of improving rabies treatment facilities, it altered the police regulations on dog control, providing for the impounding and destruction of strays, and the enforcement of special measures in areas and at times of rabies outbreaks. It was realised that the control and eradication of the disease were possibilities in an island community. Controls on the importation of dogs into Great Britain were introduced by an order made in 1897, when a form of house quarantine was required. Unfortunately, rabies was re-introduced into the country as a result of one or more pet dogs being smuggled in on a returning troopship at the end of World War I. There were 319 rabies outbreaks, all but a few of the cases being in dogs. Muzzling orders were enforced, and the disease was eradicated again in 1922. 1928 brought the legislation enforcing 6 months quarantine for imported dogs and cats, the quarantine period to be passed in approved kennels. From that time until October 1969, no case of rabies occurred outside of quarantine premises. Several times there was a large volume of protest mounted by pet lovers to have the quarantine period shortened, or abolished, for it seemed that the threat of rabies had passed, and new generations of dog owners had forgotten the fear of rabies. Those interested in exhibiting dogs at shows were, and perhaps still are, especially keen to have free exchange of dogs between Britain, USA, and Europe for the purpose of stimulating competition in the show ring. The dramatic consequences of the case of rabies at Camberley, Surrey, in October 1969, when a group of children was at dire risk of being bitten by the rabid dog, Fritz, re-awakened rabies awareness amongst the British public. During the period of the disease's recession due to quarantine enforcement between 1922 and 1969, 26 animals died of rabies within quarantine premises, and one dog was destroyed at the request of its owner and subsequently found to have rabies.

Pasteur-type vaccines unfortunately had unwanted side-effects, so work on vaccines continued. A vaccine produced by Semple and containing phenol was available for the trea ment of His Majesty's Forces in the 1920s. In 1927 it was resolved at the League of Nations conference to vaccinate annually all dogs in rabies-infected countries. In 1938 a report issued by the Pasteur Institute at Kasauli, India (a country in which rabies is common, due to the large populations of pet and stray dogs and shortage of doctors and vets) mentioned 20,000 people had received anti-rabies treatment in one year, with a fatality percentage of 0.33. In 1940 two American research doctors isolated rabies virus from a Miss Flury, transferred it to bird embryos and produced an effective living vaccine for use on dogs. This vaccine caused side-effects in far fewer dogs than had the ear ier vaccines. Another breakthrough came in 1950, when antibodies to rabies were first produced in sheep and rabbits and removed to make serum. This could then be given to patients exposed to rabies, as an adjunct to rabies vaccine. At the time of writing there are many vaccines and antisera available for use in animals and man, and a very effective, very safe vaccine for the protection of humans against the disease is now approved and obtainable by British doctors.

The Pasteur treatment with vaccine made from the dried spinal cord of infected rabbits remains the basis of modern protection against rabies, but scientists are continually seeking to refine the material used in the vaccines so that it may generate less side effects and may also stimulate antibody production more quickly. The vaccines developed by Semple, an English doctor working in India about 1911, have probably been the most widely used of all. Semple vaccine was prepared from the brain tissue of adult rabbits and sheep which had rabies virus injected into the brain, but the major advance in technique was that these were inactivated or "dead" vaccines, the infected brain tissue having been treated with carbolic acid. Unfortunately, all vaccines made from the nerve tissue of adult mammals may contain a factor which destroys the coating sheath of the spinal cord in the recipient, giving partial paralysis of a muscle or group of muscles, showing in the patient as facial twitching, mild spasm, or possibly incontinence. The course of 14 repeated doses of vaccine is likely to produce an allergic response in one patient out of 1,400, and in 15% of those who show allergy, the outcome may be death as a direct result of the vaccine and not the disease, so Semple vaccines cannot be used as preventative treatment, only for post exposure when the risk of rabies itself is greater than the risk from the vaccine. The injections are large in volume, very painful to put in, and the course consists of 14 daily injections, plus three booster doses which are larger still. The only site which will accommodate such large injections is the abdomen and the buttocks. A dog breeder, bitten by a dog imported from Africa in 1959 writes: "I had 10 cc of vaccine injected into the behind for two days, then 3 cc and 4 cc alternately under the skin of the abdomen for 18 days. By the end of this there is not one square inch which does not hurt, and it takes about six months for the discomfort to wear off."

Inflammation at the site of injection is quite common, but in view of the risk of death from rabies, this method of treatment is acceptable in many countries. With Semple vaccines, detectable circulating antibody appears within 15 days in at least 80% of patients. Another vaccine used widely in South America and Russia derives from immature mice under 10 days old, but it has proved to have no better safety record, producing in some patients acute nerve inflammation and ascending paralysis. Suckling mouse brain vaccines are not licensed for use in Britain. Duck Embryo Vaccine (DEV) is a suspension of tissue prepared from the whole infected bird, not just the brain. Human Diploid Cell Vaccine (HDCV) is now the vaccine recommended by the Department of Health and Social Security for pre-exposure vaccination in Great Britain, and it is now available to those who by nature of their work are at risk. It is also now approved for post-exposure vaccination. Most patients will show circulating antibodies in the blood after a course of this vaccine. Minor unpleasant reactions to duck embryo vaccine are quite common, but potentially lethal reactions are rare, so DEV has been passed for use wherever the much greater danger of exposure to rabies exists.

A great deal of research has gone into improving techniques for manufacturing vaccine for other viral diseases, and this work is available for use in developing an anti-rabies vaccine both as a preventative for animals and humans, and as a treatment for humans after a bite has taken place. Cell culture vaccines made on hamster cells provide a killed vaccine for use in dogs and cats. This vaccine is used on every dog and cat which enters quarantine kennels in this country, being given by a veterinary surgeon on arrival and the second dose 14 days after. Every phial of vaccine, containing one dose for dog or cat, is controlled by the Ministry of Agriculture, Fisheries and Food (MAFF), and all phials issued must be accounted for. A veterinary surgeon in private practice may vaccinate a dog which is being sent or taken abroad to a rabies indigenous country, but he will have to order the appropriate amount of vaccine and return it if for any reason it is not used, and the veterinary surgeon will require to have a sight of the Kennel Club export pedigree for the dog or cat in question. Rabies vaccine is stored under light refrigeration; it could quickly become useless if improperly stored. The cost of anti-rabies vaccination for a dog is now between £8 and £10, and the animal must have a booster each year, in a country where rabies is present, unless live vaccine is used with its attendant risks.

If rabies occurs in Britain, and by nature of the outbreak MAFF see the need to declare a Rabies Infected Area, it might be necessary to vaccinate all dogs and cats within that area, at the expense of the country and free to the owner. The vaccination would be carried out by appointed veterinary surgeons working at designated vaccination centres.

In France, thousands of cattle in the "rabid" areas are vaccinated annually with a combined immuniser against foot-and-mouth disease and rabies. In 1974, it was estimated that one million cattle had these shots. Neither of these diseases is endemic in Britain, so cattle innoculated in this way are not allowed to be imported here.

Cost of Vaccines for Human Use

Duck Embryo Vaccine costs £3 per dose in a course of 14 doses. Human Diploid Cell Vaccine, licensed in January 1977 for post-exposure use as well as pre-exposure, will cost £15 for each dose. The pre-exposure course is two doses; the post exposure will need six or eight shots depending on the location and severity of the bite. Human Immune serum used on the wound will cost another £15 or more. Treatment of post-exposure cases will be under £50 each case with the less well regarded Duck Embryo Vaccine, and over £100 with the newer and safer Human Diploid Cell Vaccine, both amounts without calculation of administrative costs.

Several cases are treated in Britain each week, mainly of people who have been bitten abroad, but also workers in quarantine kennels and the transit station at Heathrow airport, where the kennel staff frequently unpack, feed and water animals which are delayed on their forward journey.

There is always rabies somewhere in the world. At present only Britain, Australia and New Zealand, Scandinavia (except for Denmark), Cyprus, Portugal, Japan, Malta and Hawaii are assuredly free. Rabies re-invaded Denmark in September 1977 and invaded Italy in February 1977 (after seven years freedom). Within land masses where no sea barrier exists, the rabid animal is no respecter of international frontiers. Once rabies is established, it is very difficult to keep it from spreading, the disease ever aiding its own transmission when the furious form causes animals to run over long distances, biting other animals indiscriminately. In different areas of the world, rabies is spread by a variety of animals. In India and Sri Lanka, the wild and semi-wild dog is widely infected, biting thousands of people every year. In the Middle East, wolves are the vector, in South Africa the mongoose, and in the tropical areas of Central America, the vampire bat is the dangerous animal. In USA, the skunk is probably the most important wildlife reservoir, rabid skunks having been known to attack cows, horses and domestic dogs and cats. As the skunk does not usually kill its victim the disease is progressively spread. One domestic cat, bitten by a skunk, was known to have attacked and bitten its owner, and three farm dogs within an hour, so rabies spreads very quickly in such a situation, particularly when taken in its furious form. America also has a very large permanent stray dog problem, with fairly large numbers living totally unowned, not returning to any home at night.

All over Europe, rabies, is being conveyed, mile by mile, by the wild fox. Sylvatic rabies, in wildlife, has now encircled Paris with multiple cases at Beauvais, 110 kilometres inland from the Channel coast. Twenty-five per cent of the departments of France are presently affected with rabies. In these unfortunate areas all dogs must be on a lead while on the street and dogs must wear muzzles; and other pet livestock must be kept indoors. Systematic fox hunts are being organised but the possibility of stopping the relentless spread of rabies looks hopeless. Even in countries where rabies is present, the disease can subside, being transmitted very slowly where wildlife is scarce, so that no cases may be seen for months or even years, engendering a mood of false security. Rabies is alleged to pass in three year cycles, with peak epidemics killing off a lot of animals and then a low residual phase occurring when no clinical cases are seen, but when any species of wildlife gets numerically low, nature seems to take a hand in bringing the females into oestrus more frequently, or increasing litter size, so that within a year or two the population is back where it was. In Britain, we have a very high fox population, more than enough to support an outbreak of rabies, and to spread it country wide if it was not recognised quickly. Foxes are found almost throughout Great Britain, and now we have the urban fox, verging on suburbia, living under garden sheds and breeding in summerhouses not twenty miles from Central London. During 1977 a Sussex farmer trapped 75 foxes in a 200 yard stretch of his land, a well used fox run, and this only 10 miles inland from the coastal strip where the risk of a smuggled animal getting loose is felt to be high. The fox is a common sight in car headlamps after dark and fox corpses are found littered on the roadside, for many of them are the subject of traffic accidents. Although the price of £8 paid for an unspoilt pelt encourages trapping, the fox population explosion continues at an alarming rate. The fox living in built up areas is extremely difficult to eradicate . . . an overgrown garden with dilapidated sheds and a warm compost heap may harbour ten or more breeding foxes living off wild birds, pigeons, dustbin waste, insects, and fruit and vegetables. There is now an epidemic of sarcoptic mange among these suburban foxes, which is being passed on to pet animals and from them to humans, this being a precusor and warning of the situation likely to prevail if rabies ever infiltrates the British fox population, which must be at least as high as that in France. Many people feel that a fox destruction campaign should be made now ahead of any rabies outbreak but MAFF officials have decided not to risk the loss of public sympathy with the rabies awareness campaign. Equally if not more important than this "loss of public sympathy" are the economics of such a campaign which would have to be throughout the whole country and would need to be a continuing commitment. Experience in Europe has shown that, after decimation (by rabies or organised destruction), foxes are never eradicated and after two or three years the fox population is back to its previous level. While it would be practicable, and contingency plans do exist, to destroy the foxes in a limited infected area to prevent the spread of rabies, and then permit the area to be repopulated from the surrounding clean areas, a prophylactic countrywide campaign would be not only prohibitively expensive but also of little lasting value. The fox population is specially thick in Wales, where they constitute a great nuisance to farmers at lambing time, but in the Forestry Commission plantations, the fox is a useful member of the staff, keeping down the rodents which would otherwise nibble at the bark of young trees, and also serving as a natural cull for the wild deer, by taking the young fawns of about 5 lb in weight when they are only a few days old. Deer are born in late May, just when the fox cubs, born in March/April, are the biggest charge upon their parents, and very demanding of food. The young roe deer, deposited by its dam in light undergrowth for several hours at a time while she browses, makes an easy kill for the dog fox out foraging for its young.

The pattern of countryside living, both in Europe and Britain, has changed radically in the 20th century. The 19th century was the great age of game-keeping, when the nobility in their country houses took great pride in inviting kings and emperors to shoot over their land which was immaculately kept with plenty of sport available. Large numbers of outdoor staff were kept, and it was the keeper's pride to display a line of vermin, and a fox brush or two, to prove that he was doing his job in keeping the land clear of predators so that the pheasant and partridge, snipe and grouse could flourish. Then in the course of two World Wars, the pattern of life altered: gamekeeping became, as it is now, a dying art, and altered to a do-it-yourself enterprise for business executives; a different type of person was recruited to fox hunting, those that enjoyed the hacking round the roads rather than the chase, and for many hunts it is the fox which is now the master. Public opinion has turned against hounds making a kill. We live in a faint-hearted world over-saturated with the idea of conservation. Even in France, where the fox is the deadly rabies-enemy, there has lately been founded a Society of the Friends of Foxes, committed to preserving them.

The World Health Organisation Expert Committee on Rabies recommends vaccination of dogs as a preventative measure against rabies in countries where the disease or the immediate threat of it exists. They suggest that if dogs are immunised, even if they are suspected as rabies contacts, they need not be killed, but need only be re-vaccinated and kept under close surveillance for three months. The further recommendations are that puppies are vaccinated at three to four months, with a booster a year later, and that cats should be vaccinated annually. In Europe there is available a combined vaccine which protects dogs against distemper, hardpad, leptospirosis and rabies (Medivac, Hoechst) and this is the protection method usually used for newly purchased puppies. Dogs and cats given preventative vaccine show no side effects at all; they are never deliberately vaccinated after exposure to rabies. Many countries have regulations demanding the annual vaccination of dogs over six months old. Dogs are given an identity card which is stamped each year when the dog is vaccinated. In Spain, a country where rabies was rare until 1975, veterinary surgeons notify the names of owners and identity card numbers of dogs to the municipal health authorities who can tell at any given moment whether a dog has received its due innoculation. Dogs wear an identity medal to show that they are licensed and registered with the municipal authority. A dog not wearing a medal, or whose owner cannot show that one has been applied for, is taken to the municipal kennels and destroyed after three days. If the owner claims the dog in that time, it must be then registered, anti-rabies protection given, and a big fine paid to secure its release.

In Belgium, compulsory anti-rabies innoculation for all dogs, cats and other pets in the southern half of the country was ordered in June 1976 after a total of 250 cases of animal rabies had occurred south of the Meuse. There had been no human deaths but 300 people had to be treated at the Pasteur Institute in Brussels.

In October 1977 some forty thousand dogs in Southern Jutland, near the Danish/West German frontier were vaccinated against rabies after reports of rabies cases only a few miles over the border in Germany. The first case of rabies in Denmark for seven years was confirmed in a fox caught near the West German border in September, and by the end of 1977 a further six cases in foxes had been confirmed.

The German/Polish border has not been entirely free of rabies within the living memory of people who are adult today. Dogs are always exercised on the lead and muzzled, but until recently most of the rabies cases were in wild animals with few human fatalities. A small number of rabid domestic pets are much more dangerous to man than many cases in wildlife. In Germany, only vaccinated dogs may be entered at dog shows, and all imported dogs must either be vaccinated or have a health certificate saying that they come from a region free of rabies.

In Switzerland, dog vaccination is compulsory and dogs brought from other European countries to shows must also have been vaccinated.

In Canada the population of red fox and striped skunk is very high, and rabies is widespread in these creatures who also infect the timber wolf. The last fatal case in humans was in 1967, when a four-year-old girl died after being clawed by a rabid cat, although she had the Pasteur treatment. Her death was thought to be due to her extreme youth, or perhaps an inability to respond to vaccine. According to a vet practising in Canada, most pet owners ensure that their dog and cat is vaccinated at least once every two years against rabies. The vaccination is not mandatory, although free clinics are provided. It is not usual in Canada to vaccinate horses and cattle, although it is in these latter animals that most cases in domestic animals occur, the figures for 1975 being 74 cases of rabies in dogs, 73 in cats, 280 in cattle, 40 in horses, 38 in sheep, 14 in pigs and four in goats, this for the province of Ontario alone. For the same period, 658 cases were reported in foxes, 187 in skunks, eight in wolves, 18 in bats and 10 in other species. The high incidence in cattle is due to their vulnerability to bite from the fox when they are lying down at pasture. The cats and dogs affected with rabies are usually those living in rural areas.

Rhodesia has compulsory vaccination of all dogs at three months old, with boosters at one year and five years. At the same time that they are vaccinated, the dogs are tattooed in the ear with a year mark, as a check to inspecting authorities. Vaccination is free to the dogs of the black population, and heavily subsidised by the government for others. In 20 years one veterinary surgeon had only seen four rabid dogs, two with the dumb form and two furious, but as in other countries, those who have seen rabies emphasise that cases do not always follow the textbook form. Injections are put into the dog's hindleg and there are no bad reactions.

Rabies is endemic in Nigeria, dogs being considered the reservoir of infection. Control is by immunisation of owned dogs and destruction of strays. Flury strain vaccine is used, at 3 months old and again at one year, with annual boosters where there is high incidence of rabies.

There has been some desire expressed for anti-rabies innoculation to be available to dogs and cats in Britain, in advance of any outbreak of the disease. Owners have said they would like to feel their animals were protected, and a nucleus of dogs and cats already vaccinated would certainly lessen the burden on the veterinary profession in the event of a rabies outbreak, especially if it was in a highly populated city with many thousands of pets coming within the disease area. We already have quite a number of dogs and cats in this country which have been through quarantine, and so have been vaccinated, and there must also be a number of animals which have been protected prior to export to rabies countries which have in the end not left Britain. The Minister of Agriculture, in agreement with the Royal College of Veterinary Surgeons and the British Veterinary Association announced in June 1976 that elective vaccination should not be introduced because, to be effective, at least 75% of the dog and cat population would have to be vaccinated. The only way that this could be achieved would be through a multi-million pound compulsory vaccination programme which would not be justified at present. Veterinary surgeons are mindful of the fact that only about 50% of our dog population is immunised against distemper; despite many publicity campaigns it seems impossible to increase the proportion of dogs protected beyond this level. An anti-rabies vaccination programme for the fortunate dogs of owners who could afford it might well lull the public into a false sense of security so that there was less vigilance regarding the observation of the import and quarantine regulations. It is noticeable that the most frequent alibi for those caught smuggling a dog is that it has been vaccinated, so that they believed quarantine to be unnecessary. People tend to put unlimited faith in the efficacy of vaccines, especially if they have paid for them, but rabies vaccines, like every other kind, cannot guarantee protection for every animal. The other point made, and a very effective one, was that a vaccination programme, particularly if it did not cover all animals likely to be affected, such as colonies of feral cats, could render the speedy identification of rabies more difficult if it should come in from abroad.

There is also the question of the cost of rabies vaccine, if it were available in advance of an outbreak of the disease. At £10 to £15 for each animal, it would mean a class distinction for those owners who could afford to have their pets protected, against a disease which they have not got and may never get, and those owners regarding their animals with equal affection, but without the money to spend on something not immediately necessary. There is also feeling among veterinary surgeons that they could be open to a charge of profiteering if they encouraged clients to get their animals protected and then, year after year, as we all hope, it turned out that there was no case of rabies in UK. One also suspects that owners of vaccinated dogs might allow them to run loose with impunity, or might be tempted to take them abroad on holiday and smuggle them back in again, believing their dog could not possibly have or transmit, rabies.

As long as Great Britain remains free from rabies the Government, acting on the recommendation of the Ministry of Agriculture, Fisheries and Food, has no intention of permitting voluntary vaccination. Thus, anti-rabies vaccination of animals is not allowed in this country, except for animals being exported to countries where regulations require it and for dogs and cats in quarantine, where it is mandatory in order to provide an additional safeguard against the unlikely possibility of accidental cross-infection. Although vaccines have improved there is no known vaccine which can guarantee complete immunity against rabies. Much depends on the individual animal's health status, differences in quality of the types of vaccine available, the varied response of individual animals to the vaccine, and on where the bite occurs and the amount of rabies virus absorbed should the animal subsequently be bitten by an affected animal. To permit the vaccination of "native" animals in a rabies-free country would be wasteful without providing a real safeguard; it could undermine confidence in and support for the Government's proven policy of import control and quarantine, and create a sense of false security which might induce some pet owners to smuggle who otherwise would not.

The World Health Organisation also recommends a policy of import control and quarantine for rabies-free countries. The success of this policy in Great Britain can best be judged by the fact that in over fifty years only two cases of rabies have occurred outside quarantine, although twenty-seven animals developed the disease in quarantine over the same period. Both these "out of quarantine" cases were in imported dogs which had completed their six months quarantine. In addition, a rhesus monkey, mported for medical research in November 1965, died in January 1966 from rabies. At that time primates were not covered by the rabies quarantine legislation.

There are on record many cases of rabies which have occurred in spite of vaccination. In this country, a dog which died of rabies in June 1968, while in quarantine, had been vaccinated twice in the country of origin in 1967; the only domestic cat to die of rabies in quarantine since 1922 had been vaccinated; and in the last case of rabies in this country in 1970 (out of quarantine) the affected dog had been vaccinated on three occasions before importation.

In the event of compulsory vaccination of dogs and cats or other prescribed species becoming desirable as a control measure in an infected area, Government contingency plans exist for carrying out such a programme quickly and comprehensively. These plans include provision of sufficient approved vaccine, syringes, etc. within the necessary time scale, as well as the organisation of vaccination centres, the plans for which were formulated jointly with the British Veterinary Association. The cost of vaccination in an affected area would essentially be borne by the Government.

In the dog and cat, rabies anti-bodies are not evident until two weeks after the first anti-rabies injection, so these pets will be vulnerable for that time in the event of an outbreak. Occasional failures in vaccination may be through poor technique, or because the vaccine had lost all its properties at the time of use through poor storage temperature or time, because the animal was already incubating the disease, or because it was a non-reactor.

Animals other than dogs and cats may be immunised. In America skunks, as well as being one of the chief wildlife vectors of rabies, are also sold as pets. After vaccination they may break down with rabies, which they were probably already incubating, so in some American states their sale as pets is banned. In Britain dogs and cats will be injected under the skin of the neck and there is no record here that there are bad reactions to this method.

For human rabies prevention and treatment, the outlook improves all the time. The newest vaccine, prepared on human diploid cell culture, embryo lung tissue being the medium, is being developed in France, and is already being used here for people especially exposed to the risk of rabies, such as quarantine station workers, veterinary surgeons and animal attendants at the transit hostels at London Airport. This vaccine, known as HDCV, is being made at the Institute Merrieux, Lyon, France, and it was by the kindness of this organisation that enough vaccine was donated to protect the 114 contacts of the two rabies cases treated in London hospitals in 1976. Work has been done on this vaccine for 10 years, and it is now thought that we have available a vaccine as pure as modern scientific processes will allow; a vaccine free from foreign protein and yet producing high rates of antibody in response to quite small doses, so the dreaded 16 shots in the soft underbelly may be a thing of the past. The amount of vaccine needed is very small, and is given in two shots, 28 days apart, giving ample time for any skin reaction to wear off between the injections, which are put into the skin in the shoulder area, or into muscle. Even this greatly improved vaccine, which had a trial in Britain by 35 volunteers during 1975, is not entirely free from side effects, although none of them are serious or incapacitating. Sixteen volunteers who were given 1.0 ml of the vaccine intramuscularly experienced the least trouble, three said they had pain and felt ill after the first injection, and five had headaches. After the second injection, four felt ill, two had headaches and two experienced wheezing and difficult breathing. These volunteers were not segregated in any way, so it is likely that they may have caught other mild viral infections, influenza and colds at the same time. Nineteen volunteers who received much less vaccine, only 0.1 ml into the skin, had many more local reactions, nearly all reporting redness at the site of the injection after the first and second shots. Some complained of swelling and itching, aching, dizziness, headache and abdominal pain with diarrhoea and vomiting, but none of the symptoms were bad enough to keep the volunteers from work and all reactions had cleared up 10 to 14 days after the vaccination was completed. Clearly, anti-rabies protection is not very pleasant to receive, but considering the protection it offers, it is well worthwhile enduring these minor disabilities.

All the volunteers who tried this vaccine had high levels of anti-rabies antibodies in the blood after the first injection, and by completion of the course, all had far higher levels than with duck embryo vaccine (DEV). It has been authoritatively stated that no case of human rabies has occurred in people known to have had rabies antibodies in their blood serum at the time they were bitten, so it would seem likely that these

35 volunteers had acquired protection against rabies. In the future, more work will be done to see how long the antibodies persist, and what effect booster doses will have, should they appear necessary.

The Institute Merrieux also donated vaccine to treat the contacts of the two rabies patients who died in London hospitals in 1976. As one of the patients repeatedly had active rabies virus in his saliva, the need to protect all those who had been in contact was urgent, and the number amounted to 114, counting doctors, nurses, auxiliary staff and the plane crew which brought one of the patients to London. They had to be protected so quickly that there was no time to embark on a conventional schedule of vaccination, and as the numbers were large, supplies of the vaccine available were limited. The contacts were put on three different vaccination schedules. In the first they had 0.1 ml of vaccine intradermally into the upper arm, and into the thigh on Day 0, a method which produced very good amounts of antibody (although not as good as those on Schedule 2), and antibody was present very quickly. This method of vaccination is very convenient, since follow-up visits will not be necessary, but a booster dose at 21 or 28 days after the first would greatly reinforce the response and prolong the persistance of antibody.

Schedule 2 vaccinates received 0.1 ml innoculation on days 0, 1, 2 and 3, and those on Schedule 3, had 0.1 ml on days 0, 3, 7 and 14. On Schedule 3 the responses were slower, but in the end, antibody levels were higher than those in people receiving Schedule 1. Schedule 2 responses were not as quick as Schedule 1, nor as enduring as Schedule 3. Side effects of vaccination included redness, itching, and hardening of the area around the injection site but all the symptoms were mild and did not cause any absence from duty. It was not possible to find rabies antibodies in any of the subjects until three days after the initial injection, but in every respect the amount of antibody, the speed of production and the lack of discomfort for those treated makes HDCV a great improvement on previous vaccines which needed to be given in very large doses. These two trials have proved that 0.1 ml, a very tiny amount, is enough to give protection. In itself this poses a minor snag as the small dose requires special skill to administer, but it is likely that this anti-rabies vaccine will only be available routinely at Public Health Laboratories at London, Cardiff, Newcastle and Liverpool, where trained staff are available to administer the innoculation. In the event of a local outbreak of rabies, it is likely that supplies of vaccine for human treatment would be sent to a hospital in the area. In view of the cost of vaccine, it is not likely that immunisation of humans would be widely undertaken; pre-exposure treatment would be confined to those having active contact with suspect rabid animals: the dog wardens, police, ministry officials and veterinary personnel. When considering post exposure treatment for someone who may have been in contact with a rabid animal, the following criteria would be applied:

1. Was the patient actually bitten or did saliva from the suspect animal come into contact with broken skin?
2. Was the suspect animal captured and attempts made to confirm that it was rabid? If it is possible to capture the suspect animal, the appropriate virological examination can be carried out at the Central Veterinary Laboratories of MAFF at Weybridge.
3. Was the suspect animal behaving in an abnormal manner at the time of the incident?
4. What was the species of animal involved and where did the incident take place?

If this information is given to the Divisional Veterinary Officer of the Rabies Section of the Animal Health Centre of MAFF at Tolworth, Surrey, he will be able to give an expert opinion on the probability of the suspect animal being rabid.

So much time, over 10 years of costly research, has gone into the development of the new vaccine that it is inevitably expensive. The vaccination course costs between £15 and £20 if administered privately, but it is available on the National Health Service for people who are at special risk by reason of their occupation. At present this means people who work in zoos, customs officers and police in very vulnerable coastal areas, as well as quarantine kennel staff and the veterinary surgeons who supervise quarantine kennels.

In the summer of 1976, a number of veterinary surgeons, members of the British Veterinary Hospital Association, visited the Institute Merrieux at Lyon, France, where a large range of vaccines against foot-and-mouth disease, equine influenza, swine fever, distemper and cat enteritis are made as well as the new HDCV against rabies. The most striking thing about the research institute was the efficiency of organisation which enables the factory to produce in the heart of a large industrial town, vaccines against some of the most deadly viruses known to man, in conditions of total safety. The Institute was founded as a one man laboratory by Charles Merrieux, son of a pupil of Pasteur, but has now developed into a massive research and production complex. The factory is a series of buildings within a building, the jacket consisting of passage ways around the outside and through the centre of the complex, with separate sections for each vaccine production line, entered only through shower and changing rooms leading into an area under constant negative pressure of air. This avoids any possibility of organisms escaping in the event of any accidental breakage of any of the glass panels which form the walls of the production compartments. These are so arranged that once the employees enter, they have no need to leave until the end of the working day, canteen and other facilities being provided within the inner skin. Vaccine production is largely in huge stainless steel vats, holding hundreds of gallons, but it is not likely that HDCV is on maximum production yet.

Veterinary surgeons, their nurses and lay staff have been willing volunteers to test the new vaccine and record side effects, but for obvious reasons, clinical trials on those who have been bitten by rabid animals are almost impossible to conduct, for no one in this deadly danger could have treatment withheld, or be given a placebo, as is usual in trials of drugs. The best that can be done is to treat bitten people with the new vaccine and record the success rate. The latest figures involve 45 people in north-east Persia, who, between June 1975 and January 1976 were bitten by six rabid dogs and, even more dangerously, by rabid wolves which ripped them around the throat and head. After only six injections of vaccine and one of rabies anti-serum, all the patients recovered satisfactorily and show no paralytic or other serious side effects up to two years later.

HDCV is licensed in UK for pre- and post-exposure treatment. Although the possibilities of the use of HDCV are cheering, it must be remembered that the total number of recipients in France and in other countries to which l'Institute Merrieux has donated vaccine amount only to a few thousand to date. Much more data will be required before comparative merits of this new vaccine can be established.

When a person has been bitten by a rabid animal, an attempt to provide instant protection is made by injecting immune serum obtained from a person or animal which has high anti-bodies against rabies. Immune serum is also swabbed right into the bite wound in an effort to neutralise the rabies virus at source. The standard serum available in most parts of the world, including this country, is prepared in horses and cattle, but there is always the risk that the human body will reject the foreign protein. Now that more human volunteers are being immunised with HDCV it is probable that they will be able to donate human immune serum, which will not provoke unpleasant reactions in the bitten patient. Veterinary students at the teaching colleges will be asked to volunteer to be immunised and then to donate sera, as the response is best in the young and fit human. We know that the bite of a rabid animal does not always transmit the disease, and also that correctly administered protective measures do not always prevent development of the disease, but experience over the years has shown that it is always best to get treatment. An investigation recently carried out in India has shown that whereas 56% of untreated people who were exposed to rabies developed the disease, the incidence was only 7% in those who were vaccinated.

Unfortunately, the cost of producing HDCV will always be high, largely because the embryo lung tissue cells are relatively inefficient in their production of the virus, so its cost may preclude its use in developing countries where rabies is very widespread, and religious beliefs forbid the eradication of wild and stray animals which remain the vector of the disease.

Although vaccination of pet animals is usually successful and without incident, a recent report (August 1976) from a veterinary surgeon in Kenya indicates that two dogs died as a direct result of vaccination. However the disease was rife in the area at the time, so there is no conclusive proof. Dog No. 1 was a young male Jack Russell terrier, which had been vaccinated with live anti-rabies vaccine about four months before. He was brought to the vet because of intense itching and eczema in the neck, around the site of the vaccine injection. The dog was quiet to handle, but when allowed to run around, twisted its neck downwards in a frenzied attempt to rub the sore place on the floor. The dog was hospitalised, fed and watered, both of which it could take easily. In the morning, the dog was noticed eating its own faeces, and the owners said it had been irritable with other dogs. Only 30 minutes later, the dog began to attack its aluminium feeding bowls, ripping the metal up with its teeth, causing salivation, and swelling of the tongue which from then on protruded from the mouth. The dog died 24 hours later.

The second dog in the report was innoculated in the neck with anti-rabies vaccine also four months before it was brought to the vet on account of itching in the neck, which was twisted to the left, with tongue protruding. The dog was amenable to examination, but in view of the previous case, a tentative diagnosis of rabies was made. Three days later the animal became aggressive and attacked its cage; the day after, it died in the dumb form of rabies. The veterinary surgeon went on to say that in the 15 rabid dogs he had seen in recent months, these two were the only ones which showed itching in the neck and wet eczema at the site of injection, although itching at the site of a rabid bite wound is often reported in horses. Negri bodies were not found in the brain of these two dogs, and the vet felt that the cases were highly indicative of rabies caused by the vaccine and not by infection from other animals. At the time these dogs were vaccinated, an anti-rabies campaign was being conducted in Kenya and several hundred dogs were vaccinated, so it is unlikely that there was anything amiss with the batch of vaccine, leaving open the possibility that individual dogs sometimes react badly to immunisation.

Chapter 5
Modern Defences

Quarantine

The British Government's aim to keep rabies out of Britain is based on the strict control of importation of animals, with the exception of those coming from Northern Ireland, Eire, the Channel Islands and the Isle of Man, but if there was an outbreak of rabies in any of those areas, quarantine restrictions would immediately be applied. Animals which have come from overseas and arrive in this country via Ireland and the Channel Islands are subject to the six months quarantine stay, and it must be emphasised that these offshore territories are extremely conscious of their duties in this respect and very much resent the implications sometimes made that they form a "back door" way in for rabies to reach the mainland. Dog fanciers and veterinary surgeons in the Channel Islands are particularly worried about rabies, as some uninhabited rocky islands between Jersey and the French coast are visited as picnic places by both French and Channel Island families in the summer time. Therefore there is, in theory, the opportunity for French and British dogs to meet. The island of Jersey is very well served with anti-rabies posters and notices, the island slogan being PERIL, "Prevent the Entry of Rabies into Island Life".

British importation and quarantine restrictions were made more stringent following the Waterhouse Report in June 1971, after the Camberley and Newmarket cases of rabies, and three deaths of animals from rabies while in quarantine kennels in 1969. Immediately after the Camberley outbreak, when there was a strong suspicion that the incubation period for rabies might be longer than six months, or might have been masked by anti-rabies innoculation done abroad, the quarantine period was raised to 12 months, but this was subsequently returned to six months, and backed by vaccination on arrival in this country. There have been no deaths from rabies within quarantine kennels since 1970.

The fines for illegally importing an animal have been increased several times since then. A smuggler convicted in the Crown Court of a deliberate offence faces an unlimited fine as well as up to a year's imprisonment. The Criminal Law Bill which came into force on 8 September 1977 raised the fine on summary conviction to £1,000 plus costs. The fine represents far more than the cost of quarantining even the largest dog for six months, so there is little incentive in trying to evade the British law in this respect.

The Ministry of Agriculture, Fisheries and Food is well aware that some well known people may think they are above the law, so a watch is kept on gossip columns and news items in the papers about stars of stage, TV and sport. Quite often it is said that such people are devoted to their animals and could not travel without them, or that they mean to come back to settle in Britain with their whole family and their pets. Although these may just be publicity stories, the Ministry often sends a polite note with leaflets about quarantine regulations, so that there can be no misapprehension.

The Rabies (Importation of Dogs, Cats and Other Mammals) Order 1974, No. 2211 as amended in 1977 from HM Stationery Office gives the current regulations. The order covers all warm blooded animals except farm stock and some other grass eating animals, for example, camels, hippos and antelopes which are not considered significant vectors of rabies, but even these animals are subject to control if they have been in contact with species subject to quarantine.

A licence to import an animal into Britain must be obtained in advance, when the applicant will be sent details of the quarantine arrangements and a list of approved quarantine kennels and also of carriers who are specially authorised to transport animals from the point of arrival to the quarantine station. Only authorised carriers may do this, the owner cannot take his pet to the quarantine station in a private car. On receipt of the completed form, the official procedure is to check that a place has indeed been reserved in an approved quarantine kennel, and if all is in order, a licence to import, valid for six months, is issued. Among the instructions sent are warnings to land the animal in a properly ventilated container of suitable size and strength, with bars that are nose and paw proof. Two or more animals belonging to the same owner and normally living together may come in together and be kennelled in pairs, and a bitch may be accompanied by her unweaned pups, or a queen by her kittens. Animals may only arrive in Britain by certain designated ports and airports, and since February 1977 all these listed places are required to provide secure holding facilities for the care of animals awaiting onward shipment, those passing through Britain, or those whose transport to quarantine station is delayed.

The Prescribed ports are:	Dover (Eastern Docks)
	Harwich (Navy Yard Wharf)
	Hull
	Liverpool
	Hoverport, Ramsgate (Pegwell Bay)
	Southampton
The Prescribed airports are:	Birmingham
	Edinburgh
	Gatwick
	Glasgow
	Heathrow, London
	Leeds
	Manchester
	Prestwick

Only in exceptional circumstances such as if an aircraft or vessel is diverted in the interests of safety may an animal land at any other place. London Airport has a superb new animal receiving and holding centre, architect designed to high standards of safety and comfort for animals, and equipped with the most modern cleaning and ventilation devices. This hostel, built and run by the City of London, was opened in February 1977.

An animal which is passing through Britain on its way to another country must remain within the confines of the port or airport while awaiting onward transport, and may only be moved about the port or airport by an authorised carrying agent. From March 1st, 1977 more stringent rules were applied to labelling of crates of animals passing through our airports, and a tightening up of the identification procedure for the animals contained in boxes.

If the delay in onward transport involves a wait of more than four hours, the animal must be taken to authorised holding premises where there will be facilities for letting it out of its travelling box, providing food and water if thought necessary. The staff at the Animal Quarantine

Station at London Airport now cope with this work, their guests at any one time ranging from reptiles through dogs to elephants. All animals coming into the hostel must be strictly isolated from each other, and in normal times, any animal passing through Britain should be exported again within 48 hours, but in times of bad weather, delay may inevitably be longer.

Animals arriving for quarantine in Britain are usually met at the airport or at the dock, by the licensed carrying agent. The owner may not deliver the animals to the quarantine kennels in a private car or by any other means. For this reason, animals should be off-loaded in a strong container of suitable size, with paw and nose proofed bars. On arrival at the quarantine premises, every dog and cat must be vaccinated with anti-rabies vaccine, without regard to any vaccination programme which may have been performed overseas; and a second dose of vaccine will be given 28 days later. The only exceptions to the vaccination course are any dogs and cats which may be coming in for research establishments where vaccination might interfere with the purpose of the work for which they are to be used. Such animals go to special holding stations and are not kept at quarantine kennels which take cats and dogs, or other small pets. Vaccination of quarantined animals was brought in after the Camberley and Newmarket rabies incidents, when there was some suspicion that rabies might be passed between animals while actually in quarantine. Before that time rabies vaccine was positively banned in Britain, and even animals going to rabies-established countries could not be protected before they left these islands. For the first 14 days of quarantine each imported animal is strictly isolated, no visiting is allowed, and the MAFF/DAFS advice is that every effort should be made at the kennels to keep each batch of new arrivals in one block, and that batch is to be treated as a unit throughout their stay in quarantine. Up to three dogs, or three cats belonging to one owner, may be kennelled together although dogs and cats are always kennelled separately. In some ways this is considered inadvisable as it is not so easy to detect deterioration of morale, or behaviour indicative of oncoming illness, if dogs or cats are kept in a group.

Quarantine kennels are run quite differently from ordinary boarding kennels. Although holiday boarding may be provided by the same business, the two enterprises must be kept entirely separate, the quarantine kennels must have a separate entrance, and the staff must not be interchangeable with those looking after native British dogs and cats in for short term boarding. In no circumstances must an overflow of holiday boarders be put into the quarantine division of the kennels, or vice versa.

Quarantine kennels are specially licenced by the government, the licence renewable after inspection. The kennel must be under the direct supervision of a qualified veterinary surgeon, who is responsible to MAFF or the Department of Agriculture and Fisheries in Scotland for the safe custody and strict isolation of each animal in the kennel throughout its period in quarantine. The veterinary surgeon must be satisfied that the standards of those who work in the kennels, and the upkeep of buildings and fences fulfills government requirements, and the vet alone bears at all times responsibility for everything which happens at the kennels. About half the quarantine kennels in Britain are owned by veterinary surgeons, with lay personnel as day to day managers, while other kennels are in lay ownership under strict veterinary supervision. However the kennel is owned, the veterinary surgeon responsible, or his deputy who must be approved by the Ministry, must visit the kennels every day Monday to Saturday, and on Sunday also if necessary, and he or she must make a weekly report on all the animals in the kennels to the Ministry.

Quarantine kennels are designed to minimise the spread of disease, so they are built in small self-contained blocks within a tall reinforced boundary fence from which no dog or cat should be able to escape. It is usual to allocate staff to each block, so that they have permanent charge of the animals there throughout their stay, and get to know them really well. Affection and care on a continuing basis from one group of staff does much to alleviate the stress of boarding for pet animals, and a very good relationship will build up over the weeks between the animals and those who look after them, this closeness not only keeping the animal happier, but also helping the attendant to recognise any departure from normal behaviour which may indicate that the dog or cat is becoming ill.

The boundary fence of the quarantine kennel must have only one entrance and exit, which must be wide enough for a van to enter, when bringing newly imported animals in, the yard gates being closed while the van is unloaded. At the new London Airport holding premises, there is an electronically operated alarm system which closes all doors automatically, for use in the event of animals breaking out of their cages while being unloaded. Within the normal quarantine premises there must be treatment rooms, and washing and feeding facilities, and an incinerator for faeces and soiled bedding, so that no quarantined animal, or anything appertaining to it, needs to go outside the perimeter fence. The internal surfaces of the animal's living compartments must be covered in a hard impervious surface as least as high as the animal can jump, so that walls cannot become impregnated with saliva. Cats may be housed in pens two tiers high, but dogs must have a walk-in kennel. Not even the smallest breeds may be housed in the battery-hen type cages into which they have to be lifted. All aspects of the buildings and runs must be planned with a view to preventing animals getting close to each other or even coming within spitting distance when they are in exercise runs or being led past other kennels in the corridors. The Waterhouse Committee investigation found that one of the most vulnerable situations in quarantine kennels was the use of communal exercise runs, it having been the practice to take each dog to the run separately, but immediately after the previous dog had left it, and sometimes water bowls and toys had been left in the runs for all the dogs to use – water bowls containing saliva being a possible means of transmitting rabies virus. The Waterhouse report advised that individual runs should be provided for each kennel, thus saving the opportunity for animals to meet as staff took them in and out of the communal runs, and also eliminating the risk of dogs licking up saliva, urine and faeces produced by other dogs which had recently used the run, and preventing them mouthing other dogs' toys and bones. Bearing in mind that the capital outlay to provide individual runs would be very great, a time allowance was made for the improvements, the proposed date for the new standard being September 1979, by which time all quarantine kennels must have individual runs, all newly built kennels since 1971 conforming to the new standard automatically. After 1979, any kennels unable through financial stringency, or lack of room, to provide individual runs are advised to revert to normal holiday boarding for British resident dogs and cats. While communal runs at quarantine kennels still have to be used, only the same group of dogs should use each run, being put out to exercise in the same order each day.

Animals undergoing quarantine may have their own individual bowls, toys and grooming equipment, but these items must not be used for other animals, nor must any of the animal's "luggage" leave the quarantine kennel until the end of its stay. All hair clippings and uneaten food must be destroyed. It follows that quarantine kennels are usually sited in isolated places, well away from houses and towns.

Once in the kennels, dogs and cats must keep to the same living compartments for the whole of their stay, only being transferred if absolutely essential by permission of the supervising veterinary surgeon, who must keep a record of any change of compartments. Very rarely, if the owner is totally dissatisfied with the management of the kennels, or perhaps by reason of the transfer of the owner's home to the other end of Britain, a move between quarantine kennels may be made, with Ministry permission, but transport may only be done by licensed quarantine carrier. In exceptional circumstances a licence may be granted for the temporary removal of a dog or cat to a veterinary clinic for surgery, should it be necessary and not practical to perform within the quarantine kennels.

A case history is kept of each animal in quarantine, with dates of arrival, dates of vaccination, name and batch number of vaccine and any illness the animal may have or accidents which may befall it, including illicit meetings with other animals. The integrity and good faith of all kennel staff is very important in this respect, as the consequences of any lapse in observance of the daily rules could have great significance, not only to the animal concerned and its owner, but also in tracing back any disease outbreak which may occur later. Where an accidental meeting between animals, or inadvertent use of the same feeding dish is admitted and recorded, a disease outbreak may be accurately attributed. Where there is carelessness and concealment, a whole new quarantine regime or banning of animals from certain countries might be instituted, in the belief that our quarantine precautions are not yet strict enough.

In addition to the visits of the supervising vet six times weekly, spot checks are made by government veterinary officers at about three monthly intervals, and a visit is always made to attend postmortem examination of any animal dying while in quarantine. The head and neck of the animal must be sent to the Central Veterinary laboratory at Weybridge for examination for possible rabies infection, and the rest of the carcase must be destroyed on quarantine premises. Any companion animal to the one which died must be retained in quarantine at least until the results of the tests are known. The veterinary surgeon must make a report in his weekly return of any deaths or illnesses, and even of animals being in a low state due to fretting and pining, for misery of this kind could just possibly be indicative of the early stages of rabies.

The duties of the supervising veterinary surgeon extends beyond the health of the animals to surveillance of the kennel staff, recording any incidents of biting and scratching by animals, seeing that wounds are properly disinfected and notifying the local Medical Officer of Health of any such incident. Where the animal inflicting the injury is due for release within 15 days, consultation must be made with the Ministry to see if it would be prudent to defer release. Any escape or theft of a quarantined animal must be reported immediately to the police, the local authority and to the Ministry.

Quarantine kennels are virtually a closed community, never open to public scrutiny. Only the veterinary superintendent, his deputy and his staff, the veterinary officer of MAFF or DAFS in Scotland, and the kennel proprietor and his workers are allowed within the boundary, with the addition of authorised visitors to the dogs and cats. Visits may be made to quarantined animals after the first 14 days, while the primary vaccination takes effect, not only by the owners, but also by their appointed friends and agents, but only by permission of the kennel proprietor. Permission will obviously be withheld if the animal shows signs of aggression and illness, or if the visitor creates unrest in the animals. The visitor may groom the dog, play with it, and bring it titbits, but while they are making the visit they must be willing to be locked into the run and kennel with the dog. Any toys or possessions which are brought for the pet must remain with it and cannot be taken away again until the animal has completed quarantine. In the owner's interest, any biting or scratching incident, however slight, should be reported at once. Opinion is divided about the wisdom of visiting pets while in quarantine. Nearly all kennels have some visiting hours on six days of the week, some being unwilling to allow visitors on the Sunday when the veterinary surgeon does not make a routine call. Many people feel that it is asking a lot of a pet animal to see its owner for a short time infrequently and then to settle back into kennel life, and often it takes some time for the kennel staff to console the animal and get it to settle into kennel routine again after a visit. Almost certainly, the visit is more for the comfort of the owner than for the pet, and in many cases it would be best to let the animal settle down and only to make enquiries by telephone.

If a bitch or a queen arrives in quarantine with suckling young, the pups or kittens must be weaned off the dam by the time they are 10 weeks old. The young ones are then confined in groups of three or less for the remainder of the period of detention.

Quite often show-stock bitches and queens are imported already pregnant, this being a useful way to bring in a new blood line by an overseas sire. If the pups or kittens are born 14 days or more after the dam has been vaccinated it is assumed they will receive rabies antibodies via the colostrum or first milk from the dam, and will not require vaccination themselves if they leave quarantine before they are three months old. If they remain in quarantine beyond this age, they will be given their first injection at three months and a second shot 14 to 28 days later, if they are still in quarantine. If pups or kittens are born within 14 days of the dam receiving her first injection, it cannot be assumed they will receive maternal antibodies, as they may not yet have formed in the dam, so the young ones must be vaccinated at one month old, and again one month later, and a third time at three months, if they are still in quarantine kennels, the third vaccination being necessary because of the uncertain level of antibodies transmitted by the dam, particularly if she has been vaccinated before overseas. Similarly, very young pups and kittens imported without the dam may need three injections, and these young ones must complete the full term of quarantine; pups and kittens born while in quarantine may be released only with special permission of MAFF or DAFS.

All vaccination must be with a type of vaccine approved by the Ministry and used in accordance with the manufacturers' instructions. Certificates of vaccination must be issued to the owner, and copies lodged with MAFF or DAFS, and also one copy retained at the quarantine kennels. Dogs and cats may not be mated while they are in quarantine, nor may semen be taken from a male for the purposes of artificial insemination, and no canine semen may be imported from countries where rabies is present.

The number of pets being put through British quarantine kennels is rising all the time. In 1949 under 2,000 dogs and cats were legally imported. By 1960 the numbers were around 2,500 dogs and 500 cats, and in

1969 there was a total of almost 4,000 dogs and 1,000 cats. In 1976, 4,250 dogs and 1,600 cats were imported legally, and 138 other mammals, these travelling in batches and probably destined for experimental work. Many of the dogs were show stock as there is now considerable interest in bringing over European Sheepdog breeds and gun dogs from Iron Curtain countries. A conservative estimate of the cost of importing a dog in 1977 would be £400, covering quarantine stay, collection from point of entry in quarantine kennel's transport, and veterinary fees for statutory injections; the freight charge for carriage from country of origin and travelling box being extra. There is very little variation in the charge for a small dog as basically the main costs are the same except for food, which is a minor item. A cat would cost around £250 to import now. Fees are payable monthly in advance, and the vaccination fee is an additional charge on the first months' bill.

At the end of six months, or the prescribed quarantine period, the dog or cat must be removed from the kennels. The owner is given a card detailing the procedure to be followed if rabies symptoms are shown, and the address to which the dog or cat is released is kept on file. It is surprising how well most animals endure their quarantine stay. It is not at all unusual for a dog imported by an exhibitor to come straight from quarantine to take prizes in the show ring, winning compliments for being in excellent condition, but sometimes a young dog will be rather shy of traffic and noise after having spent a comparatively big proportion of its life in seclusion. The lack of daily walking exercise seems to be much better tolerated than our pets would have us believe, for no dog in quarantine is taken for walks, and yet they come out looking very fit indeed.

Some people returning from long stays abroad send their pets on ahead so that the quarantine period is nearly over by the time the owners arrive here. This programme has much to recommend it, the only disadvantage being that there may be no one in this country who has complete knowledge of the dog's or cat's history should illness arise. Horses are not required to undergo quarantine, and there is a fairly large traffic of show jumpers, racers and bloodstock between France and Germany, Britain and Ireland. The reasoning behind the free travel for horses is that the horse is a very limited vector of rabies, and it is only very high quality stock, supervised by experienced personnel which will be travelling between countries in this manner. Before a horse is brought to Britain it must have a full clinical examination by a veterinary surgeon, and be given a certificate of good health, and the premises on which the horse has been kept for the previous three months must be certified as free from rabies. The horse may only travel with similar animals, horses, mules or donkeys, and no pet dogs may be brought with it as familiars. The importer or the British owner is handed a card, on the arrival of the horse, detailing the symptoms which might lead to suspicion of rabies and the procedure to be followed if such symptoms occur.

Farm livestock, cattle and pigs may not be imported at all, save only for a few specially authorised imports for breeding purposes. These animals, which must not have received the combined foot-and-mouth and anti-rabies vaccine within one month of their exportation, must come only from a farm which has been free of rabies for the preceding six months, and the herd from which the cattle come must be certified free of disease. Farm animals are quarantined under direct government veterinary supervision before they are exported, and for a similar length of time after landing in Britain.

Zoo animals may be directed into accommodation approved by MAFF at urban zoo premises, provided they are kept in escape proof cages, and separated from other animals and the public so that no disease risk exists. Zoo animals may be put on exhibition during the quarantine period.

Mink and other animals bred for fur may be imported straight to breeding farms provided that the new batch of animals is isolated, and kept in secure approved quarantine accommodation.

The number of travelling circuses and the use of animal acts in them has declined rapidly in the past few years, due to public antagonism for such performances. Lions, tigers and zebra bred in captivity in British safari parks are available for training so there is no need to import or exhibit foreign circus animals.

Mammals which are allowed to be imported without quarantine restrictions include: dolphins, whales, porpoises, seals and walrus, duck-billed platypus, elephants, manatees and aardvarks. These animals are unlikely to be a source of rabies infection, and they are unlikely to be confused with any other animals for which quarantine regulations do apply.

Chapter 6

The Vector of European Rabies: The Fox

In Northern Europe rabies became apparent in sled dogs during the 1930s, causing a lot of deaths among them, but it was not immediately diagnosed, probably because the low temperature made the symptoms atypical, and also because there were no human cases. Sled dogs normally fight a great deal among themselves, and their handlers are used to evading bites; they are also habitually well covered in thick clothing which would render them less vulnerable. Until 1939, rigorous and continuing efforts of the public health authorities in France, Germany and Scandinavia meant that rabies had been eliminated from the domestic pet, and that wildlife, especially the red fox, was kept to minimum numbers. World War II disrupted the control measures, and hunting and shooting parties were suspended, never to return again on the same scale. Everything combined to make a fox population explosion possible. There was ample waste food in the wake of army camps and troop movements; the fox population "never had it so good". In France, the deserted buildings and labyrinths of corridors of the Maginot line have proved to be ideal lairs for thousands of foxes, these animals being particularly adept at taking over existing cover for their own use. Foxes are not pack animals; they spend much of the year alone or in pairs, only living in a family group of dog fox, vixen and cubs for two to three months of the year after the cubs are born in March/April. British foxes do not all belong to the same sub-species. *Vulpes vulpes crucigena*, the more common red fox, weighs around 18 lb as an adult, about the size of a small terrier, with its brush, or tail, being half the length of its body. There is also a larger variety, with a greyish tinge to the fur, similar to the Scandinavia foxes, *Vulpes v. vulpes;* these stronger animals are said to be descendants of foxes with great stamina, imported from the continent to give hounds a better and longer run. This type of fox is found in Scotland, and the higher parts of the Lake District.

The fox is somewhat of a parasite among mammals, an opportunist in taking over the habitations of other animals. The hill fox prefers broken country, rock scree, peat beds and cliff ledges where it can curl up and sleep in the sun, retreating in the shelter of rocks when there are people about, and moving around mostly at night. The lowland fox is again not domestically minded, and it prefers to find ready-made accommodation. A large rabbit burrow will suit, a field drain, a badger sett, or it will just lay up in a patch of gorse. Badger setts will become vacant more frequently in the future, as a campaign of gassing is being carried on in the West Country, as badgers have been found to be passing tuberculosis to cows at pasture where herds have been TB free for some years. Such setts are sealed off and resealed if opened. The fox will have many homes within its territory, some of which it has had to abandon owing to its habit of defaecating within its den, making it, after a time, uninhabitable. Artificial fox earths constructed in hunting country are always made low at the back, so that fox cannot squat to foul the den. Food is brought back to the resting place, and left in an untidy litter of mammal and bird remains, as well as evidence that quite a lot of bilberries and blackberries are eaten in autumn, but the fox is primarily a meat eater, so meals can be spaced at long intervals, giving plenty of time to move around, to play, and to kill for sport rather than need. Foxes can also digest starch, and may pillage open barns where grain is stored, but in Britain now the smart fox finds easy living around litter bins in country parks, around the dumps at motorway cafeterias, the refuse left by campers and caravan hot dog stands, and the open tips where household rubbish is deposited. The fox is the ugly predator of the carcases of pet dogs and cats, given euthanasia by the vet, which have to be put on open tips in some areas because this is the only means of disposal available for those owners who cannot bury their pets.

The fox follows its daily trail rather than to break new ground; about 3 miles is the average territory for one adult, marked out by urinating against posts and trees as a dog does. When the territory is suitable, and some shelter available, the fox lives above ground for most of the year, only two months being spent in the earths while the vixen rears her cubs. Just at the time that foxes will be mating in December and January, very big wild boar shoots take place in Germany and Poland. The quarry is driven by dozens of beaters on to the guns, and this will disperse the foxes, aiding the spread of rabies. On the Spanish border, riders and hounds drive boar up to the guns, again widely scattering other forms of wildlife. In Britain, all such sporting activities would be suspended when there is an outbreak of rabies in a particular area, so that diseased animals are not artificially scattered.

In January, when mating is taking place, the eerie cry of the vixen can be heard at night, with the answering short bark of the dog fox. Once paired off, they are said to mate only once, tying like dogs and their wolf relatives, and the dog fox is alleged to be faithful to one vixen for life, remaining celibate if the vixen is killed. The cubs are born underground, blind, deaf and helpless, in late March, early April. The average litter size is five. The young suckle for 8–10 weeks, coming to weigh about 1,250 gms at 10 weeks. They get their second teeth at 16 weeks, very similarly to the dog puppy, but reach adult size sooner, at about six months. Rabbit is their commonest food, after that, sheep, birds, insects, rats, mice and voles and shrews, the fox liking variety in the diet and preferring to live where a wide range of food is available. The dog fox brings food for his young family, and teaches them to play, fight, stalk and kill, sometimes bringing back half killed prey so that the cubs may practise a kill. In the autumn the cubs begin to disperse to seek territory of their own, for they never remain in a family group for the winter. Autumn would be the peak time for spreading rabies, for the young foxes travel widely seeking territory of their own. A MAFF survey made in the Welsh hills, carried out by attaching a radio transmitter to the collar of a fox, showed that the distance travelled by a dog fox in its search for living room might be as much as 32 miles, but is probably nearer to 10 miles on average. Vixens seemed usually able to settle within 4 miles of the place where they were born, but dog foxes only found a place an average of eight miles away. During this search they cover a lot of ground, and have a great deal of social contact with other young foxes, and probably fights with adults in dispute about territory. The fox is an excellent spreader of rabies, because it normally enjoys carnage and shows no reticence about biting when in good health. In a state of furious rabies, foxes will attack cattle, deer, sheep and goats. They have bitten tethered dogs, and dogs within their own gardens. They will take kittens, and bodies of cats killed on the road, so it is likely that the rabid fox would chase and bite the domestic cat. In terms of danger to humans, the pet dog or cat which is bitten but escapes is a great hazard, particularly if the bite goes unnoticed in the animal's fur. The dog or cat which is killed by a rabid fox can do no more harm, but owing to the compulsive desire to run during the furious phase of the disease, the fox is likely to bite and pass on, rather than stay to finish off its victim.

In France, 47,000 foxes were destroyed in one year, and £14 million are spent annually on control measures. The first case of fox rabies in that country was reported in March 1968, to reach a total of over 2,100 in 1974, giving a total of 5,708 confirmed cases of fox rabies in six years.

In France an intensified campaign to reduce the fox population is carried out, chiefly by gassing in the dens during the breeding season, using hydrogen cyanide, and by paying a bounty to hunters on production of a fox brush. France has also passed a law allowing entrance to private property for the purpose of exterminating foxes for the public good, and in July 1976 an order was made in the parts of the country where rabies was most strongly established, to round up all cats which were straying and destroy them on the spot, except that dogs were given a 48 hour stay of execution to allow owners to claim them, if they have been vaccinated. Pets will never again be allowed out on their own in the north and eastern corners of France, after this salutary lesson on pet keeping by the government.

A few rabid domestic animals are much more dangerous in terms of human rabies than hundreds of wild animals, so in many countries, pet animals are vaccinated against rabies voluntarily, or in Switzerland, compulsorily. The precaution pays off, for in Switzerland, only 2% of emergency treatments for humans were needed through the bites of suspect rabid dogs, whereas in Germany, 21% of cases in humans demanding emergency treatment are through dog bite, and there have been five deaths in humans from this cause. In the Federal Republic of Germany, it is not uncommon to find a rabid fox dead in the woods. Some restrictive measures would then be imposed, dogs having to be kept on a lead outside towns and cats not being allowed to run free within a certain distance of villages. If many carcases are found, or a rabid fox appears in a town during the day time, a "rabies endangered district" is declared; dogs and cats have to be confined to houses, dogs only exercised when on a lead and wearing a muzzle, and any dog or cat running free is killed, without further warning. Dogs and cats require veterinary permission if they are to be taken out of the district, and even when moved, they are subject to the same restrictions for at least three months. But still rabies spreads across Europe.

In Germany, bounty is also paid for foxes shot, but co-operation by field sportsmen is low, and killing the animals off has not helped a great deal as it is found that individual foxes cover greater territory searching for mates, so spreading the disease more widely. Where a vixen is deprived of her cubs, through gassing in the dens while they are young, the vixen has been found to come into heat and produce another litter at a time when it was not thought that there would be any foxes in the dens, so these second families were reared successfully.

In Britain, a survey of the methods of fox control mentions shooting, gassing, poisoning, snaring, trapping and hunting, but if sylvatic rabies were to be found in wildlife, hunting and shooting would almost certainly be forbidden, as any method which would tend to harass the foxes and spread them out would defeat its purpose. Gassing might be effective in early spring, if the breeding earths could be found. This might be the only method of control suitable for the urban fox living close to houses. Snaring would require experienced personnel and is a slow process. It is possible that the gin trap, banned for some time now in England, might be brought back, if used only by official and experienced personnel. The remaining method is poisoning, and this would meet many of the requirements of a campaign to deplete the fox population. Foxes will readily take bait which would be laid unpoisoned for ten days, to accustom the fox to feeding in certain places, and then poisoned bait would be laid for two days. A campaign using poison could be mobilised very quickly and could be carried out with the help of armed service personnel and other officials who have not had any special woodsman experience. MAFF have special powers to use strychnine in this campaign, which would only be conducted in the face of a rabies outbreak, when no pet animals should be loose to have the opportunity of taking this bait, which is an almost instant killer. Promising progress is being made in research to find an alternative poison which is humane, quick acting, without the undesirable persistency of strychnine, and to which an antidote is available if needed.

Two methods of fox control which might be developed in the future also use bait, frequently chicken necks, but this time they would conceal either oral anti-rabies vaccine, or a contraceptive pill to reduce breeding potential. Neither of these methods would be of any immediate use in the event of an outbreak in Britain when the aim will be to clear a limited area of foxes, but not other wildlife, unless there is evidence that other species are becoming vectors of rabies, so that the outbreak may be quelled very quickly, thus preventing rabies from moving into the country as a permanent menace. In December 1977 The Nature Conservancy Council made a grant of £22,000 to the department of zoology at Bristol University for a project of investigation into the role of the red fox in rabies-wildlife transmission.

Chapter 7

Rabies in the Animal Species

If our greatest fears are realised, and rabies does come to Britain, how will the first human case be recognised? Will someone arrive at a doctor's surgery, complaining of a headache, an overpowering depression, and an uncomfortable feeling in the throat? British doctors have had almost no opportunity to diagnose rabies, so it is not likely that the disease would come to mind, unless there was clear history of a suspicious dog bite, but in any case, the rapid worsening of the symptoms would mean that hospitalisation would become necessary within a few days, and then specialist opinion might connect the unhappy patient with rabies. To find human rabies as the first case would be a very sad thing, with the almost inevitable death sentence. Rabies is a notifiable disease all over the world, so once suspicion or positive diagnosis is made, in animal or man, the health authorities and MAFF must be told. Immediately, a tracing procedure would be set in motion to find out where the infection came in, and what and where the other contacts had been. The circumstances would be more sinister if the animal or the human patient had not been abroad, for it would point to some undiscovered domestic animal having, or having had, rabies in this country.

The biggest injury that the animal smuggler can do to us all is to illegally import a dog, which subsequently becomes rabid, and then to turn it loose, into the countryside, or into a town, to wreck its terrible way to death on other animals and perhaps humans too. The smuggler would no doubt be in great fear of the consequences of his crime, and therefore might be tempted to take a line of least resistance and divest himself of a sick animal, or to let it go during the furious phase of rabies. This is the way that rabies came to Amsterdam in 1962, when five people and a lot of different animals died, and 500,000 dogs and 165,000 cats were compulsorily vaccinated within two months, costing the country a great deal of money, all because someone brought a little white dog from North Africa, and then turned it loose.

If rabies is first found in wildlife, it may turn out that the disease has been in the country for some length of time, undetected until foxes begin to attack cattle, or domestic animals. Sylvatic rabies could then have spread over a wide area, needing a great slaughter campaign of both diseased and healthy wildlife before we knew we were clean again. The uncontrolled domestic cat, and the semi-wild feral cat colonies could well be the transmission link between sylvatic rabies in foxes and rabies in pet animals.

It may be that the warning bells will ring when a vet sees a dog in his surgery, or a cat on a house call, which have at least some of the rabies symptoms. Again, if the suspicion deepens contacts will have to be traced, and perhaps the owner will have clues to give about a bite, or a fight with some free running animal. The long delay between the incident, and the manifestation of symptoms is one of the big hazards in tracing back rabies contacts.

In the Camberley and Newmarket outbreaks, it was very fortunate for us that the history led straight back to quarantine premises, and that the vets consulted had rabies experience, so there was no spread of rabies at that time.

Rabies in the Dog

The course of the active phase in the dog lasts from three to eight days, but infective virus may be present in the saliva up to five days before the obvious symptoms are shown. There is production of virus during most of the time the animal is visibly ill, but virus has left the saliva immediately before death. The early signs in animals vary a lot, and may be scarcely noticed, but restlessness, nervousness, unexplained fear, lack of appetite and vomiting have all been recorded as the first disturbing signs. A definite change in temperament is always suspicious; while a quiet dog becoming irritable, and excitable fits the classical picture of the disease, an aggressive and fierce dog which suddenly feels affectionate and sentimental may be giving the warning. In countries where they live with rabies, a change of mood in an otherwise difficult dog is not always attributed to a triumph of the trainer's art. Slight signs of paralysis are important to notice, it may be as little as a drooping lower eyelid, a lameness or the carrying of one limb.

The nervous habit that some otherwise sound dogs have of leaping up to catch invisible flies is another sign of brain disorder which becomes more significant in a rabies situation if the dog never behaved in that way before. The dog may hide away from bright light and may even attack its owner if attempts are made to drag it out from under the bed, a favourite place of refuge. The dog incubating rabies will be easily startled by loud noise and may bite itself at the site of the original bite wound. There may be muscular tremors, when the dog holds itself rigid, shaking all over. The dog will almost certainly appear anxious, frightened of its own feelings, terrified of the strangeness which has overcome its familiar world. The pupils of the eyes may be wide open, but not holding any expression, giving the traditional mindless stare so often shown in the old pictures of rabid animals. The lips curl back to reveal teeth and gums, the tongue hangs from the half open mouth which the dog cannot close, and saliva, which cannot be swallowed through paralysis of the throat, is drooled in large quantities. When the head is shaken, the saliva is thrown widely in droplets, and that saliva is dangerous, should it get into a cut on the hand, or into the mouth or eyes. It must be a frightening and piteous situation to see a well loved family pet producing the symptoms of rabies, for the instinct will be to help and comfort the dog, especially in the quieter phases, but in the true sense of the word this could be a fatal thing to do, and even if protected by vaccine, the suspect rabid animal is best left to trained personnel to handle, for no vaccine is 100% efficient.

Many of the symptoms of rabies are the same as those of much less terrible diseases. Distemper gives discharges from eyes and nose, and makes the dog hide away from light, as indeed any sick animal tends to do. Any dog that is in pain, perhaps from an injury in a road accident, will hide away and offer to bite anyone who forcibly tries to handle it. The bitch undergoing a phantom pregnancy will show an unexpected change in temperament, and will offer to bite those who try to remove her from her invisible puppies. Some types of poisoning will cause the dog to collapse suddenly, with foaming at the mouth and convulsions. Epileptic dogs will have muscle tremor and shaking, and any kind of non-transmissible brain infection or tumour will give alteration in the appearance of the eyes, and demonstration of anxiety and fear.

A British veterinary surgeon, Mr R. Minor who is working in Kenya, reported in the *Veterinary Record* on a series of 19 dogs brought to his surgery for a variety of illnesses, all of which proved to be rabies from tests made after death. Mr Minor comments that the clear-cut division between dumb and furious rabies so often mentioned in text books was not a feature in his cases as most of his dogs were able to be handled. The tables below, reprinted by kind permission of the Editor of *Veterinary Record*, show the presenting signs and those developing before death:

TABLE 1: Numbers of dogs with specific clinical signs and histories at time of presentation

Abnormal locomotion: inco-ordinate movement (2), hind limb ataxia inco-ordination (2), fore limb lameness (2), weight transfer from foot to foot (2), back arched (1)	9 dogs
Paralysis of group of cranial or cervical muscles: i.e. jaw (3), tongue (3), deglutition (2), lip (2), neck (1)	8 dogs
Conjunctival congestion (bloodshot eyes)	8 dogs
Inappetance	6 dogs
Excessive salivation	4 dogs
Itching	3 dogs
Recumbent/comatose	3 dogs
History of bite by stray dog or association with known rabid dog	3 dogs
Shivering/trembling	3 dogs
Conspicuously aggressive	2 dogs
Mildly aggressive (resented handling)	2 dogs
Vomiting	1 dog
Convulsive	1 dog
History of non-specific abnormal behaviour	1 dog
History of absence from home	1 dog

Figures in brackets show numbers of dogs within the group affected in the described manner.

TABLE 2: Numbers of dogs showing specific clinical signs during course of disease

Abnormal locomotion: inco-ordinate movement (6), impaired balance (4), hind limb ataxia (4), fore limb lameness (2), weight transfer from foot to foot (2), back arched (1)	13 dogs

Paralysis of group of cranial or cervical muscles: i.e. eyelids (6), jaw (5), tongue (4), deglutition (4), lip (2), neck (2), oculomotor (1)	13 dogs
Conjunctival congestion	13 dogs
Conspicuously aggressive/destructive	8 dogs
Shivering/trembling	7 dogs
Abnormal vocalization	5 dogs
Excessive salivation	5 dogs
Mildly aggressive	4 dogs
"Fly snapping"	4 dogs
Itching	3 dogs
Rigidity of fore limbs	3 dogs
Vomiting	1 dog
Coprophagia (eating own excreta)	1 dog
Abnormal sexual behaviour	1 dog

Figures in brackets show numbers of dogs within the group affected in the described manner.

Mr Minor's series involved 7 dogs under a year old, 5 of those being under 6 months. He comments on the high incidence in young puppies partly due to great susceptibility but also to their curiosity and to their lack of defence against attack by strange dogs.

Diagnosis, even for the trained veterinary surgeon must err on the side of caution if there is anything in the history of the animal to provide a link with rabies, but it is also sad to think that in a country where rabies is found, dogs which urgently need help for other diseases may be regarded with great caution and not attended as they are here, with every sympathy, because we have no need to fear that they may be a threat to our own lives. One of the more distinctive early warning signs is said to be an alteration in the bark, and a recognisable rabies-type howl, before any other symptoms are shown. In the last two cases of rabies outside quarantine kennels in Britain, the case in Camberley in 1969 and the one in Newmarket in 1970, we were fortunate that there was a direct tracing of the sick dogs to release from quarantine kennels so there was a stronger pointer to rabies diagnosis, and even more fortunately, the veterinary surgeons which saw the dogs had experience of rabies cases abroad, as comparatively few British vets have had the opportunity to do.

It is a little disconcerting to realise that although veterinary surgeons see examples of most animal illnesses before or soon after they graduate, very few will have ever seen a case of rabies, and so their diagnosis must rest largely on what they have read, in conjunction with the history the owner can give them. Although both the Camberley and Newmarket dogs had served their full six months in quarantine, leading to the suspicion that incubation time might be much longer, there were certain indications at that time that the regulations for the operation of quarantine kennels were not stringent enough, so that the dogs may have been exposed to infection while in the kennels. After the two incidents, an enquiry committee was set up under the Chairmanship of Mr Ronald Waterhouse, QC "to review the policy and precautions against rabies in Great Britain and to make recommendations". The report of the committee, now known as the Waterhouse report, was made in June 1971. Until this time the regulations for the operating of quarantine kennels, and the design of the buildings turned upon the assumption that it was necessary for one rabid animal to bite another. After investigation by very distinguished veterinary surgeons it became apparent that there was the possibility that rabies might be transmitted by an indirect route, that saliva might remain for a short time on gateposts or wire, or in communal drinking bowls and that another dog might become infected by licking, sniffing or drinking the water polluted in this way.

Substance was given to this theory by the fact that a dog imported from India had become rabid and died within the same block of kennels which held the Camberley dog, which became rabid after release. On the other hand, this dog, although examined and pronounced fit on release from kennels, showed the first symptoms of rabies only seven days after, so it was possible that the incubation period might have been just a little longer than normal. Another dog in the same quarantine kennels became ill about a week before its six months of detention were due to be over. The first signs of discomfort were of stiffness in the shoulder, and muscular tremors with some inco-ordination. This dog went on eating and drinking, but also seemed restless and was panting a lot. The owner requested that the dog should be destroyed, and on postmortem, rabies was confirmed. This dog had the habit in Germany of going off hunting, in an area where there was rabies in wildlife, so there was the opportunity for it to have encountered rabies only shortly before it came into the quarantine kennels. The dog from Camberley, called Fritz, was a much more protected pet. The dog lived in the officers' quarters of a British Army camp in Germany, and there had been no confirmed cases of rabies in the vicinity for four years. This dog did not run loose, and it was not possible to find any way it could have been in contact with rabies before it entered British quarantine. Fritz was healthy throughout his quarantine, and for the first few days of release behaved normally, but on the seventh day, his owner noticed that he was behaving oddly, hiding under the bed and refusing to come out. When dragged into the open, the dog seemed to be paralysed in the back legs, and it refused food and water.

The next day it seemed better, and would eat, but not drink. One can imagine that some of the symptoms might have been dismissed as a reaction to the exciting life it had returned to, after the confinement of quarantine. By the next day, Fritz was becoming aggressive, and excitable, and the owner noticed that the bark had changed in tone. By the following day, there was a classic case of furious rabies. Fritz bolted from the house, killed a cat, bit at the boots of a milkman and vanished at top speed into the rough country of Camberley Common. About an hour later, Fritz was seen getting into a taxi full of children being taken to school. This may have been a brief return to sanity, as Fritz was used to children, or he may have wanted to hide away from daylight under the seat of the car, or perhaps he was going to attack. Fortunately, in an act of great courage, the owner of Fritz dragged him out, getting bitten twice in the process, but in doing so, she undoubtedly saved the car load of children from dreadful danger, for the damage that could be inflicted by a mad dog in a tiny space among terrified children hardly bears thinking about. By this time the owner must have had a great fear that Fritz was indeed rabid, and this suspicion was confirmed by an army veterinary surgeon. Fritz was removed to a locked kennel in a quarantine station, where for two days he showed all the signs of furious rabies, a very dangerous animal indeed. The veterinary surgeon who visited him said that the eyes were dilated, and the dog refused all food and water, being found dead in its kennel just seven days after the first signs of "odd" behaviour. Fritz showed most of the typical symptoms of rabies except that, when he killed the cat, was running loose, and biting, he did not have the excess outpourings of saliva which would have been expected.

The Newmarket bitch, a terrier cross named Sessan, had been imported from Pakistan, and had also recently completed her stint in quarantine, together with a companion animal owned by the same family. Sessan became ill, over five days, with a progression of symptoms concerned with refusing food, and vomiting, but she was still drinking. She appeared very depressed and sad, and was drooling saliva. Normally, she was a great barker, but she had stopped doing that since the vomiting started, and she was producing a lot of saliva. The vet noticed that the bitch could not close her lower jaw, and in a further day or two, swallowing anything became impossible for her. The diagnosis from the early symptoms might have pointed to distemper, or gastro-enteritis, or some form of poisoning, but when the bitch became paralysed, the indication was rabies, and the bitch was taken into custody at a research establishment where she was kept in maximum security until she died, very quietly, eight days after the first signs of illness. Her companion dog was given euthanasia after the owner had discussed the position with the Divisional Veterinary Officer of the Ministry of Agriculture. Sessan had dumb rabies, and at no time was she aggressive, noisy or violent in any way. She showed no desire to run, indeed for most of her illness she was unable to do so, through the onset of paralysis, and it must be emphasised that this pattern of rabies in the dog is much the most common.

The furious form of rabies, when it occurs, is characterised by extreme activity, and the desire to run at frantic pace over very long distances, up to 30 miles has been recorded; or the animal may run in circles, holding its head at an angle, co-ordination and direction sense already being lost. This phase of compulsive activity is one of great danger, for the dog, cat or fox which runs may attack any other animals or humans it meets during its deadly progression. Depending on the amount of stress its heart will stand, the animal may go into convulsions and die in the furious phase, or it may gradually slow down as paralysis overtakes it, and die in a coma.

An mals which are confined under suspicion of rabies may attack and destroy their cages with unnatural strength. They may eat stones or cloth, and tear at wood with their teeth, howling wildly and behaving like a demented creature, which is, of course, an apt description of the rabid animal. Fear of water is not shown by dog or fox; even if they are unable to drink, they do not shy away from water in fright as the human patient does. They dog may drink water in large quantities, losing a lot from the mouth through oncoming paralysis of the jaw. Dogs and foxes occasionally will even swim across water which they find in their "furious" path. Sometimes there are periods of normality in between frantic episodes. The domestic animal which has run away may return to its home, exhausted and looking pitiful and ill. Its sympathetic owners may handle it at this stage, at great risk to themselves, if they are unaware that the animal may be rabid. The dumb form of the disease, which may be the only one shown, or may precede death after the furious demonstration, will show the dog with drooping head, the lower jaw sagging, the mouth permanently open and saliva drooling out. The growing paralysis of the hindquarters makes the dog stagger and fall about, and there is general inco-ordination of movement, the front legs gradually failing too, and the neck stiffening up. Howling will by now have stopped, but the bark may change in tone, as the throat and voice box become paralysed too, as the brain cells are destroyed and cease to be of use to the dog. Death from heart failure takes place between four and eight days after the first signs of the disease were shown. No animal that is suspected of incubating rabies, or has been bitten by an animal showing rabid behaviour, can be treated in any way at all. It is unlikely that any family would want to retain any pet, however well loved, if there was the chance that it might become rabid and a danger to themselves and the community. The only possible exception to euthanasia for the bitten pet, would be in the case of a dog or cat which had recently received anti-rabies vaccine, in the situation of a rabies outbreak; such an animal might be permitted to be put into quarantine for six months, being regarded all that time as potentially dangerous. Such quarantine would be at the expense of the owner, and it is not likely that visiting would be allowed, in the case of a pet known to be very much at risk.

Cats

The cat is more susceptible to rabies than the dog, and for humans, the cat bite and scratch may be more dangerous, as the teeth can penetrate more deeply into tissues. In the first phase of the disease, the cat may show an unusual amount of affection for its owner, but later becomes unpredictable, and vicious. When the cat bites or scratches, it is likely to hang onto its victim, rather than biting and running off, as the dog does. The cat will hide away from light, under furniture or in the dark corner of a shed, and will howl continuously, probably attacking other cats, dogs and people. As the virus causes the head and neck to become sensitive, there may be a marked fear of wind currents, or the draught from an electric fan. Excessive outpourings of saliva will be noticed, with later on paralysis of the lower jaw, the voice box, hindquarters, and finally death will put the poor animal out of its misery. It is unfortunate that the extreme danger in handling rabid animals makes it impossible to give them euthanasia even when it is realised that death is inevitable.

As in the dog, the early stages of rabies in the cat are similar to many symptoms of less terrible and more common diseases, so in a country where there is rabies, a great deal of unnecessary worry and heart-ache must be experienced when any animal falls ill. The fear that rabies might be present may lead to some degree of rejection of the sick animal, at a time when, in other types of illness, it most requires its owners care. On the other hand, the consequences of rabies are so dreadful that it would be extremely silly for any one to be a hero and out of bravado handle a rabid animal, which is at that time, however mild its normal nature, a killer.

The cat in a rabies country presents a bigger problem than the dog, because of the many colonies of semi-wild cats which live on hospital premises, factory compounds and dockyards. There is already great concern about the growing numbers of these cats, which live quite well on waste food, and are of some use to their landlords in that they keep rodents down. However, a semi-wild colony of unknown numbers of cats would constitute a focus of potential infection should an outbreak of rabies occur. In an effort to keep numbers down, there are schemes afoot to feed a contraceptive pill to these cats, and another to catch up the males and castrate them, using charitable funds for the purpose of limiting to some extent the breeding activity in the cat colonies

The predilection of cats for hiding away in places where they should not has led to more than one rabies scare in Britain. In 1977, two cats were seen to emerge from a refrigerated lorry which in theory should have been sealed since the start of its journey from the Middle East. There was much argument about the possibility of these cats surviving intense cold for so long. They were treated as rabies suspects but did not have the disease and it was concluded that the cats had the opportunity to get into the lorry after it arrived in Britain. In this, as in every other incidence of suspect rabies, decisions depend on the story told by those in charge at the time.

October 1977 brought a rabies scare to Northern Ireland, when a cat which was believed to have stowed away in a crate from Czechoslovakia escaped on to the dock at Rosslare, but returned to the ship which went on to Wexford where a posse of police marksmen finally located the cat and shot it. Tests showed that it did not have rabies, but the incident was regarded as a useful educational experience for police and port workers.

Cattle and Other Ruminants

In both America and France, cattle are the domestic animals most affected with rabies, many deaths are caused, but cattle rarely pass the disease on. The human cases attributable to cattle have been where farmers, mistaking the choking symptoms for a foreign body stuck in the animal's throat, may put their hands in the animal's mouth to explore and clear its air passage. The resultant saliva, whether the farmer is bitten or not, has the opportunity to infect him through mouth, eyes or nose if the hands are put near the face. The early signs in cattle are depression, lack of appetite and falling milk yield, which of course, are also signs of other disorders in a milking herd. If the furious form of rabies follows, the cattle will seem irritable and impatient, stamping the feet and bellowing, but in an unusual tone. There may be unusual trembling of the ears, staring eyes, tail twitching, and grinding of the teeth. Sometimes there is frenzied sexual excitement and mounting of other beasts; aggression will take the form of a desire to butt the head against fences, trees and rushing at humans – the classic "mad bull".

The dumb phase in cattle, which may follow straight after the early signs or after a furious interlude, brings on the choking symptoms and difficulty in swallowing. Later the paralysis will start at the hindquarters, when the cow will go down into a lying position on its chest, and will die with its head and throat extended forward, about five days after the first symptoms were shown. Cattle which die of rabies will be unsuitable as food animals for humans or dogs.

The course of the illness in sheep, deer and goats is similar, although sometimes the only sign may be a digestive upset followed by paralysis and death. Cattle, sheep and deer are not very efficient biters, so they are unlikely to pass the disease on except through their saliva. Herds of cattle and goats are at risk if a rabid dog, fox, or cat has been through the herd, biting them on head, nose or feet; the wild deer in our forests will be very much at risk from rabid foxes, which would not normally kill deer but seem to be endowed with extra power and aggression during the furious form of rabies. Herds of sheep, normally at great risk from free running dogs, would be an easy task for savaging by a rabid dog or fox. The seasonal incidence of rabies varies with different species, cattle having a peak in November, deer in March, after rutting but before the new generation is born.

Pigs

Pigs become very vocal when affected by rabies, they squeal a lot, attack each other and their attendants, a frantic pig being a very dangerous animal indeed. As in the other animals, many other diseases show similar signs, and in farm animals, none of the symptoms are as clearly defined as they are in the dog, cat and fox and other meat eating animals.

Birds

Poultry are said to be subject to rabies infection at least experimentally, but there is only one case on record of someone being pecked by a cockerel and requiring anti-rabies treatment, so the risk of rabies in poultry may be largely ignored. In any case, it seems logical to conclude that the chicken or goose bitten by a rabid dog or fox would die of the bite before rabies viruses had time to multiply. The same situation applies to all other British birds, but birds and gamebirds like pheasant, found dead, might have been killed by a rabid animal and so could be dangerous to handle for some hours after death, and it could be unwise to eat them, where rabies is known to exist in the area.

Rodents

Rats and mice are very susceptible to rabies. Very young mice are used in one of the definitive diagnostic tests to demonstrate that secretions like saliva and tears of a suspect case, or smears of brain tissue, do in fact carry rabies, as the mice will show rabid evidence in 21 days. Yet rodents do not appear to excrete the virus in their saliva or transmit the disease, although a World Health Organisation survey has stated that more people in the Lebanon are given post exposure treatment following rat bites than after dog bites. An authority in Malaya has stated that when healthy mice were caged with mice deliberately infected with rabies, none of the mice salivated and the rabid ones did not transmit disease to the healthy. The WHO Conference on Rabies in Frankfurt in November 1977 concluded that "rodents play no part in the epidemiology of rabies". No case of human rabies has ever been attributed to rodent bites.

Horses

Horses commonly show the furious form of rabies, using their great strength to stampede, destroy their stable and bite people during tempestuous rages. The earliest signs are refusal of food and poor appetite, depression, sweating, a facial twitch and frequent urination, all symptoms of colic or any bad abdominal pain in the horse. The tail may be held high and carried stiffly. The disease lasts only three or four days before inco-ordination and general paralysis brings about death. Horses at pasture are very susceptible to bites from dogs and foxes running madly in the furious form of the disease.

Wild Life

In the fox, badger, raccoon, mongoose and free living mink the progress of rabies is very similar to that in dog and cat, but the most marked feature in the early stages is the loss of natural fear of man, and larger animals. Naturally timid wild animals will come close to houses and allow themselves to be handled by children, at their most infective stage. Nocturnal animals which are seen around by day, fully active in a reversal of their natural habits, must also be regarded with the greatest suspicion. In the furious stage, all wild species will attack and bite human beings and animals which would not normally be their enemies. The rabid fox may even invade gardens and attack domestic animals which are ostensibly protected. In Germany, dogs kept in kennels and runs are always sited within view of the house, for fear a rabid fox should get into their runs. In Europe, it is the fox which predominates in the spread of rabies; in America skunks, foxes and bats lead the statistics.

Vampire bats (*desmondus rotundus*) are an important rabies vector in Central and Southern America, as is the fruit eating bat in USA generally, but there are no bats of this species in Western Europe outside of quarantine premises and zoos. The vampire bat is the only animal which must be imported into quarantine and remain in those conditions for life, together with any progeny it may produce. The European bats, of the species *myotis* and *pipistrelle*, have never played any significant part in the spread of rabies.

Wolves, which are a feature of the wildlife of many countries, including Canada, Alaska and the Middle East, contract rabies, but not nearly so commonly as foxes. It seems that when there is excess wolf population, skunks and other small wild animals may be caught for food and the wolf bitten in the process. In contrast to the low incidence in the animal, many people have to be treated against rabies infection from wolf bite, as their attack method is to go for the throat and face, and serious lacerations are made.

At the invitation of the Parliamentary Secretary to the Ministry of Agriculture, a small group of experts are to examine the possibilities of exterminating the 4,000 coypu rats which infest East Anglia since their escape from fur farms.

Exotic Animals

Monkeys, lions, tigers, leopards and otters are equally prone to rabies and they may infect other animals and humans.

Other Sources of Infection

It is possible in theory to become infected by eating the meat or drinking the milk of animals which are incubating or have died of rabies, but pasteurisation will kill the virus in milk, and in the sophisticated public health conditions of the Western world, the chance of getting rabies infected meat is infinitesimal, unless the meat comes from dubious source, or is poached, or found dead. The rabies virus may persist in the body of an animal which has died of the disease, for 24 hours at least, and as it is possible to become infected through the mucous membrane of eyes, nose and mouth, gloves, goggles and face masks should be worn when handling suspect carcases or at postmortem. The same precaution applies when handling freeze dried material imported for taxidermy.

Animal Bites

Although in America people have contracted rabies through breathing in the air where bats are congregated, rabies is usually the result of a bite from a rabid animal, or a lick, containing rabid saliva, on an open sore. Owing to the long incubation, the incident may be forgotten, for quite insignificant bites have had disastrous consequences.

Dog and cat bites are always taken seriously in Britain. Even if the skin is not broken, people will attend a hospital casualty department with a dog bite when a similar injury made by metal or stone would be regarded as unimportant and treated at home. There is much more blame and recrimination, and more genuine fear if a child is injured by a dog bite, than if it fell, or cut itself in some other way, and the hospital attendance, even if unnecessary, seems intended to reinforce the reproach. The Liverpool Walton Emergency Accident Unit saw over 2,000 cases of dog bite in one year, but 92% were graded as superficial, and only one case in five needed to be seen again by the doctors. In Glasgow, in the same year, 2% of casualty attendances were for dog bite injury, over half the patients being children under 14 years old, but here again, in 25% of the cases, there were only tooth-bruises, and the skin was not broken. Although there was no reference to rabies, both parents and older patients are very worried about the most trivial bite inflicted by an animal, believing animal saliva to convey tetanus, but there is no proof that tetanus arises from dog bites. Nevertheless, each case taken to hospital receives tetanus toxoid injection, as a means of maintaining the level of immunity within the population, but this ploy also reinforces the notion that dog bite injury is especially dangerous. Cat scratches can be potentially dangerous in a rabies situation, but are not, in general, so much feared by the public. Bites from a rabid cat are very dangerous, due to the level to which the sharp teeth penetrate, and the habit the cat has of hanging on, while the dog is likely to bite and run away.

In a non-rabies situation, dog bites are primarily the injury of childhood, with boys of between five and nine years old being most at risk. Bites are said to be most frequently inflicted in summer, with August as the peak month, and the timing between 2 p.m. and 7 p.m., and the majority of bites happen when children are visiting the dog's owner, so the inference must be made that there is an element of jealousy, or guarding, in the dog's aggressive behaviour, possibly feeling the owner is in some way being threatened. Dogs are possibly more irritable in hot weather, but there is also more interaction between children and dogs, and even more visiting in the summer months, so no special conclusions may be drawn from the timing. Dogs are often extraordinarily possessive, and will resent extra children touching toys and furniture even if they are absolutely reliable with the children of the household. We must also bear in mind that children make unexpected noises, and unpredictable movements, which the dog may interpret as a threat. The majority of bitten children deny that they were in any way interfering with the dog.

Half the bites were inflicted on the legs of children, but in those under four, the probability was that the bite would be on the face or abdomen, as dogs tend to spring up when they attack. In the survey made, small male dogs were the culprits, inflicting twice as many biting episodes as large dogs, and bitches. Most of the dogs were in some measure guarding house and property; the straying animal rarely feels impelled to bite unless injured or cornered with a view to capture. Of adult victims, bitten while working, postmen, paper boys, meter readers and gardeners were predictably the ones on the receiving end. Veterinary surgeons, kennel owners and people who work in grooming and trimming parlours are seldom bitten, as they are accustomed to handling all animals with the utmost caution. Dog bites will take on a new significance in the face of a rabies outbreak, and it is likely that dog owners will be expected, as a social duty, to protect other people from any possibility of being harmed by their pet. There will be even more incentive to own a well trained, good tempered animal which is completely controlled by the owner, as life will be far too difficult for those who try to keep a dog which is badly behaved. Where rabies is present, or may be present, dogs are always supervised, kept within their owner's property, and not allowed to run off. Any other sort of behaviour is asking to have rabies brought into the home.

The Risk of Rabies

Not every human being who is bitten by a rabid or suspect rabid animal will develop the disease; it is estimated that about half the people bitten will never know any more of the disease, even if they receive no treatment. How badly they are bitten, and where – head and face being the most dangerous – will certainly affect the outcome, as will the victim's state of health at the time, and the amount of virus which was present in the biter's saliva. Prompt post-exposure treatment of bitten humans keeps the number of human deaths in the Western world very low . . . in USA. where rabies is widespread, there have only been 10 deaths in 10 years among a population of 200 million, and only two of those cases involved dogs, but the cost in terms of medical care and vaccination programmes is an enormous burden on the country. In USA 30–40,000 people receive a course of vaccination against rabies every year, and the cost of medical time and facilities is estimated as 50 million dollars annually out of municipal funds. Where medical attention is paid for privately, a dog bite costs the victim 50 dollars. In France, counter measures against rabies have already cost the country more than seven million pounds.

Chapter 8

Rabies in the Human Patient

The onset of rabies, in the human patient, begins with headache, lack of appetite, a dry mouth and thirst, sore throat and aches all over . . . it could mean a bad bout of influenza, except for a tingling sensation at the site of the original bite, even though it will be by now completely healed. There may be vomiting, diarrhoea, and a worrying anxiety which persists at night so that sleep does not come. There may be a little difficulty in swallowing at first, but within a couple of days, the muscular spasms of the throat intensify, so that the patient is terrified of choking, unable to swallow saliva, or to drink at all. This is the direct result of the cells of the brain which control the neck being destroyed by the rabies virus. There is fever, but the patient fears a cool sponge, and cannot bear an electric fan switched on to create a current of air, as the muscles of face and throat are so sensitive that even the pressure of air will cause spasm. Saliva flows copiously, and the patient is constantly spitting, but dryness of the throat gives rise to a harsh cough, said to be like a bark – part of the old mystique of the illness when the patient was described as being like a dog. Localised congestion of blood cells in the brain, due to inflammation produces totally irrational behaviour, and delirium, with wild thrashing of the limbs and a desire to get free, almost to climb out of the body which must seem in the grip of inhuman torment. The patient will want to be absolutely quiet and in the dark, any sudden noise will bring on another spasm which may lead to heart/lung arrest. During the course of this phase of the disease one of the most tragic aspects is that the patient may be calm and lucid for short intervals, able to talk and to rest quietly, but able to appreciate the gross changes that are taking place and understand their cause. The calm intervals become progressively shorter, with always the dread of the next paroxysm, which will be more dreadful than the last, until the patient dies of paralysis of the lungs, or complete bodily exhaustion.

In the Western world, patients are nursed in intensive care wards, under sedation to relax the muscles as far as possible, and in the quietest possible conditions. The sound of running water is particularly banned, as it causes panic in a patient who cannot swallow but is, in the truest sense, dying for a drink. Fluid intake is supplied by intravenous drips, although so much saliva is being lost that it becomes difficult to keep the body fluid in balance. Although food is sometimes taken for a short while after drink is refused, it is preferable for the patient to be fed by the nasal or rectal route, as the fear of choking is very real.

Rabies patients are nursed in strict isolation, and all staff wear gowns, boots, gloves, hats, protective visors and masks, and they are protected by anti-rabies vaccine.

Modern intensive care units have prolonged life in patients where rabies was proved, from animal tests, to be present, and there are recently two reports of people making recovery from rabies, after having been through all the clinical symptoms, but one is said to have extensive brain damage. These are the first cases ever recorded of recovery from rabies once the encephalitis symptoms have appeared. The goal of medical research workers is to find the means of keeping the patient alive long enough for vaccine and serum to overcome the live virus.

As the early symptoms of rabies are similar to those of other virus diseases, another great boon would be a positive diagnostic test which would give early recognition of the disease, or proof that there was no rabies virus present.

At present there is no laboratory diagnostic technique which is satisfactory in all respects. In Britain, every suspect case of human rabies is examined by three methods, which are the most suitable in terms of accuracy, speed in getting the result, operator safety, cost and convenience.

Test 1

The fluorescent antibody test, known as FAT, applied to smears of brain or salivary gland tissue or impression smears from the eye, when affected cells will show in contrasting colour when looked at under a microscope equipped with an ultra violet light. The result of this test is known almost at once.

Test 2

Examination of tissue specimens, saliva and tears under microscope in a laboratory. Result in two working days. Taking fluid from the spinal cord for examination is painful in the extreme for the patient.

Test 3

By innoculation of the brain tissue of very young mice with test material from the patient, usually saliva or tears, as the taking of brain tissue would be very unpleasant for the patient. Encephalitis can be seen in the mice between one and two weeks after innoculation, according to the age of the mice. Result within three weeks.

Another test involves taking corneal smears from the eye of an animal which has inflicted a bite, for examination under ultra-violet light. There is no test which will positively state that a case is NOT rabies. At best, there can only be the very high probability that the material examined does not contain live rabies virus or rabies antigen.

Recent Rabies Cases

A pony kept at a holiday camp on the Bavaria-Austria border developed rabies, and an international hunt had to be mounted for any of the 600 people who might have ridden or petted the pony before its death . . . 10 days before being the crucial period.

In December 1976, a small white dog in the furious phase of rabies, went on a rampaging run through the city of Jerusalem for a period of 40 hours, during which 26 people were bitten, and an unknown number of animals. The dog was shot when it took refuge under a car, a marksman purposefully leaving the head intact, so that the brain could be examined in a laboratory, where tests confirmed that it was rabid. All Israel, the Golan heights and the Gaza strip are now declared rabies danger areas, and a national campaign to destroy stray dogs and cats has been mounted. Tons of poisoned meat have been procured, and already, hundreds of dogs and thousands of cats are said to have been poisoned. About 14 people have undergone the course of 14 injections necessary with duck embryo vaccine. Rabies came to Jerusalem from the Golan heights through infected foxes.

During 1976, three men died in British hospitals of rabies contracted in India and Gambia.

The first man, a student seeking religious faith in India, was admitted to a London hospital for investigation, with a history of stomach trouble which had been going on for a long time; he was thin and in poor health generally. After four days in hospital, he complained of excrutiating headache, and seemed unnaturally agitated; he refused to swallow water but could take a little food, but the symptoms alerted the hospital that this might be a case of rabies. A searching cross examination by the staff brought out the information that the man had been looking after a sick puppy in India six weeks before, and it had, at that time, scratched and licked him, although the marks were by now completely healed. He had taken no precautions against rabies. Saliva was collected for diagnosis, which proved positive for rabies, so anti-serum was given, also a transfusion of rabies-immune human plasma, obtained from someone who had been vaccinated against the disease and had made antibodies; and duck embryo vaccine was injected, but after the onset of brain inflammation and damage, these measures had no effect. Mice innoculated with the man's saliva showed signs of rabies after 15 days. Rabies virus was isolated from the man's saliva collected on the 11th day of illness, but did not appear on the second, the eighth or the fourteenth days, demonstrating the variable incidence of infection of this disease. Presumably, in a biting animal, rabies virus is sometimes in the saliva and sometimes not, producing somewhat of a roulette wheel chance of infection even from an animal which is almost certainly progressing towards death from rabies.

If the use of resuscitation equipment had not been available, this patient would have died of the massive heart attack which occurred on the sixth day of his illness. With the aid of a ventilator and intensive nursing, the patient was kept alive, through several other incidents of heart block, and also through bleeding from the stomach, due to his gastro-intestinal disability, and not the rabies infection. The man suffered from repeated episodes of choking, stimulated by any touch or movement of the neck and head. He was confused, and raving, despite dosing with tranquillisers, and he complained of difficulty in moving his jaw, breathing and swallowing. On the 11th day of illness, the spasms decreased in number and severity, and the patient seemed more comfortable; he could follow objects with his eyes, and attempted to speak. The two following days were quieter, with only a fairly mild episode of heart block. On the 14th day, surgeons performed a tracheotomy, making an opening into the windpipe through the neck to ease the breathing problems, but from then on, the man's conscious level deteriorated. On the 15th day, he became totally unresponsive, with eyes fixed open and staring, apparently not feeling any pain and not requiring any sedation or muscle relaxants. During the following week, the patient survived many episodes of heart block, until he died of a final massive attack on the 22nd day. For the last seven days of life the patient was quite unaware of surroundings and was not able to feel pain or respond at all to those attending him. Diagnosis of rabies in this case was partially obscured by the stomach trouble which the man already had when bitten, and continued to suffer while incubating rabies, and of course, through his own failure in taking anti-rabies precautions in a country where rabies is very widespread and where thousands die of the disease every year.

In the second case of human rabies in London, a man was bitten on the lip by a stray puppy in Gambia. Although he consulted a doctor he was told there had been no rabies in the area for some time, so no vaccine was given . . . but rabies is always present in Africa, and there always has to be a first case in every district. Some seven and a half weeks after the biting incident, the patient felt an odd tingling in the left arm, which by the next day had become more intense, and was spreading to the other limbs. He could eat, but found difficulty in swallowing fluids, fearing to choke. On the third day of the illness, the patient's wife ran him a bath, but he became wildly agitated, and refused to go near the water. On admission to hospital, he was still very distressed, and producing so much saliva, which he could not swallow, that a towel had to be held continuously to his mouth. Apart from mental and physical distress, examination showed nothing at all abnormal, until the patient asked for a glass of water, but when it was brought, leapt up with a strangled cry and tried to jump from the window. The consulting physician saw this episode, and immediately related it to rabies, and the man was questioned, and the story of the bite on the lip came out. Anti-rabies serum and duck embryo vaccine were given at this stage, and the patient was flown to the Hospital for Nervous Diseases in London where the best possible care could be given. All the attendants and the crew of the plane which brought the man were given anti-rabies vaccine. On arrival in London, on the sixth day of his illness, the patient was completely rational in his mind, able to give a clear account of the history of the dog bite, although he was very apprehensive, and unable to stop spitting saliva which would not pass down the throat. He began to have episodes when the lungs would not fill with air, reaching a crisis point where he could hardly breathe at all and the voice rose to a strangled high pitched scream, the lips and face becoming blue tinged through lack of oxygen in the blood. Tranquillisers were supplied by intravenous drips, but the man became more distracted, struggling violently, and the spasms could not be stopped except under massive sedation which paralised most of his body functions. Losses of saliva were enormous, over two litres a day being ejected from the mouth, causing dehydration of the body which in itself would cause death had the fluid not been replaced by means of intravenous drip. On day seven, the patient was put on to a ventilator to maintain breathing, and was connected to an ECG machine which recorded brain waves; urine was removed by means of a catheter, and the throat was surgically pierced to by-pass the swallowing mechanism. The paroxysms were entirely controlled by sedation, and all the patient's bodily functions were taken over for him, to relieve strain on the heart and other organs. The patient remained totally quiescent, and there was no response to pain, or to eye stimulation, when the lids were rolled back to see if he would respond. After three days in this state, on day ten, the sedatives were briefly withdrawn, so that the patient's state could be assessed, and there was a return of spontaneous spasms, and profuse production of saliva, but no return to consciousness. All life support measures were then returned until the 14th day, when another test withdrawal found no movement at all, no spasm, and no response to nerve stimulation, so no further sedation was given. The ECG machine reading showed a gradual decline in brain activity. The area of the brain controlling voluntary movement was out of action from day 14, and by day 20 there was no evidence, via ECG of any brain function. The patient's nominal life was maintained by a heart/lung machine until day 34 of the illness, when life support measures were withdrawn and the patient declared dead.

Although there was no doubt that this patient died as the direct consequence of rabies, rather than from any associated complications, it proved impossible to isolate rabies virus from saliva, tears, or spinal fluid and mice innoculated with these substances did not show rabid symptoms, nor did their brain tissue react at laboratory tests. It is well recognised in medical circles that rabies cannot be isolated from either animals or humans who have survived the disease for long periods. The virus had gone by the time of death, and as is usual in human rabies, no one had been bitten and the utmost precautions had been taken against cross infection, so that was the end of that transmission cycle of rabies. The physicians attending this case remarked on their inability, despite all their resources, to alter the course of the illness, by preventing the multiplication of the virus within the central nervous system.

At the postmortem, performed two hours after death, part of both lungs were found to be collapsed, and the heart enlarged, as were the liver and kidneys, the spleen was grossly heavy, and the entire nervous system of the body had been destroyed.

In both the men the incidence of bites had been quite trivial and disregarded, the patients not being treated with anti-serum in the wound or subsequent vaccine until after the clinical signs were shown, even though they were working in countries where rabies was well established. Although the thought of rabies is so terrifying, it is possible, after living with the disease for a long time, to become complacent about it.

These two patients were kept alive for considerable periods by all the resources of modern medicine available in one of London's great teaching hospitals, in the hope that the body's natural defences and the action of serum and vaccine would burn the virus out, if every assistance was given to prolong life. Treatment of rabies in less advanced countries results in the death of the patient in from two to nine days after first showing symptoms.

On 9th June 1976 a 53-year-old Indian waiter was admitted to a Manchester hospital complaining of pain and frequency of passing urine; a diagnosis of prostatis and cystitis was made and he was catherised and put on continuous bladder drainage. The man seemed to be frightened and anxious but not unduly so once treatment had started. During the night he complained of difficulty in swallowing but no abnormality of mouth or throat could be found. Next day his behaviour was noted as bizarre, at some moments hostile to the nurses, at others unduly affectionate, and there was still reluctance to drink. At mid-afternoon the patient fell out of bed in an eleptiform type of seizure and after that said he had lower abdominal pain. An exploratory operation was performed but revealed only a slightly inflamed appendix. Late that night the patient began to scream and foam at the mouth and wounded the hand of a nurse with his teeth. Attempts to give sips of water sent the man berserk and it was at this point that the attending doctors thought of rabies.

Relatives were questioned through an interpreter and it was found that the man had been in India 15 months before and there had been some reference to a dog bite but it was not clear whether the patient himself had been bitten. While discussions were being held the patient had a massive heart attack and died. The patient had spent two days in hospital in a general ward and there was great concern about infection. The bed, floor, partition and equipment were treated with chlorvos 1% and although normal high temperature washing would have been sufficient for the linen, it was burnt in order to satisfy the anxiety of the staff. Twenty-five members of the staff were treated with a course of anti-rabies vaccine. Following post mortem parts of the brain tissue were sent to Colindale Laboratories for tests in mice and a positive diagnosis of rabies was received on June 30th, 20 days after the death. Again it was only the violent refusal of water which gave the clue for the other signs of illness could have applied to much more common disease. As far as it has been possible to find out, the contact with the rabid dog must have been more than 15 months before the symptoms showed, a longer interval than is common.

A Case that was not Rabies

In February 1976 a middleaged farmworker was admitted to hospital because he had become, over the previous three days, quite unable to swallow. He was in danger of dehydration because he could not even re-cycle his own saliva. He was restless and could not sleep, constantly having to spit out saliva, as it accumulated. The patient became worse over the next three days, having difficulty in opening his mouth. Tests for a foreign body or growth in the throat proved negative, so a tentative diagnosis of mild tetanus or rabies was made by the specialist, but the patient could recall no encounter with "mad" dogs, nor was there any suspicion of rabies being in the country, and the patient had not been abroad. Treatment for tetanus was started, but there was no immediate improvement. The patients jaw was rigid, salivation copious and temperature high; he was under sedation and being fed and irrigated through a vein in the arm. After 16 days with little improvement, the patient, all the time in high fever, had a slight spasm in all limbs three times during the night, each tremor lasting two to three minutes. From then on, the patient improved, and laboratory cultures revealed that the disease was an atypical tetanus infection. Mobility gradually returned to the jaw and the patient recovered fully, being discharged five weeks after admission. This case must have looked at times extremely like a developing rabies, especially as the patient was in a hospital at a north-east coastal port where people are very much aware of their vulnerability to rabies infection through the illegal entry of animals.

First Aid Treatment

The first aid treatment of a bite from a suspect rabid animal, or where face or wound have been licked by such an animal, is to wash the site very thoroughly with a 20% solution of soap and water to remove as much saliva bearing virus as possible. After all traces of soap have been removed with plain water the newer antiseptics, Cetrimide or Hibitane, should be swabbed on to the wound. It is important at this time to keep track of the biting animal and to detain it in a safe place if at all possible; an outside lavatory or a garden shed will do temporarily. The fact that the animal is available to move to a place where it can be observed and tested under restraint may drastically shorten the period of uncertainty about diagnosis and very much lessen the strain on the victim.

The patient should then go to a doctor or hospital without delay, so that treatment may be started by putting anti-serum in and around the wound, to prevent rabies virus becoming established in a nerve along which it can travel to the central nervous system. A course of vaccinations is then started, to try to localise infection in the wound and to establish immediate passive immunity, by bolstering the body's natural defence system to produce antibodies. Immediate application of this routine treatment is proving very successful in averting the onset of the rabies symptoms.

Rabies Hysteria

Because of the terrible consequences of rabies infection, in countries where there is an epidemic and many lives are lost annually, it is to be expected that doctors will see a number of cases of rabies hysteria, a fear of contracting the disease which is almost as violent and destructive as the disease itself. The subject seems to have the impulse to wish themselves into a rabid state and to mimic the symptoms, as far as they are known, in a desire to end the suspense of waiting for true symptoms to develop. The extent to which the hysteria copies the true disease depends whether the patient has seen a case develop in a friend or relative, but it is a unique feature of this mania that the patient does not wish to be proved rabies-free. He will report to the doctor very soon after the biting incident, demonstrating symptoms which could not have developed in the time. The tendency is to mimic animal symptoms, barking, biting and running away. If the doctor tries to make any positive tests – the fan treatment of a current of air across the throat is frequently used – the patient will attack the doctor. Unable to act out a real revulsion to water, and inability to swallow, the patient will deliberately spit out water taken into the mouth. The imitated spasms are untypical, and the patient usually refuses to communicate at all, although a real rabies patient is able to talk in the early stages. Patients do recover from this nervous affliction but it takes a long time. Rabies hysteria is common in India and Sri Lanka where hundreds of human deaths from rabies occur each year, as it is impractical within the economy of these countries to undertake a vaccination programme, and stray animal clearance is not possible, owing to the religious ban on taking life.

Chapter 9
The Smugglers

How may rabies come into Britain? It is quite certain that no fox will swim the English Channel or the North Sea. More viable possibilities are that a cat or a dog may escape from a vessel in dock and mix with feral animals on land; that a ship's cat or dog incubating rabies will be exercised in the vicinity of a mooring, and will bite a British dog or cat; that a pet animal already showing signs of rabies will be turned loose on land from a ship; that an animal from overseas may stow away in a ship or container vehicle and get loose in Britain, subsequently to show rabid behaviour; or, by far the greatest risk, that an animal which has been abroad to a rabies indigenous country will be brought in secretly with human aid, in other words by smuggling, and this animal may become rabid later. It is extremely unlikely that an animal in the furious stage of rabies will be imported in any way – such an animal would be too noticeable and too dangerous to be handled. In the paralytic stage it is possible that a small animal might conceal itself in a road vehicle or ship, but in this case the disease would be almost self-limiting as such an animal would not be able to move about and spread the disease; the only danger might be to a person who tried to touch it.

There is some degree of danger that animals from abroad which are on ships in British harbours may land, and mingle with our own animals. Many suggestions have been considered in efforts to tighten up the regulations associated with visits here by foreign boats, and also with the vastly increased numbers of small boats which leave British marinas to sail towards the French coast in the summer.

It is easy to understand that it is impossible to watch every yard of our coast line, all the little beaches and inlets at which a small boat might put in for a few hours. Many boats carry dogs as companions, watchdogs and pets, and most ships will have a cat as rodent exterminator. The control of these animals while a vessel is in port is largely in the hands of the crew, for it is manifestly impossible to board and search every vessel, but Customs men and harbour masters keep a keen watch. The owner or captain of any vessel is required to sign a Customs declaration form and to confine animals on board while in port. In Hawaii, which also has the good fortune and prudence to be free of rabies, a $2,500 bond must be furnished by the commanding officer or owner of a ship, undertaking to keep the animal in security and not let it ashore while the ship is in harbour.

The Rabies (Importation of Dogs, Cats and Other Mammals) Order as Amended in 1977 states that an animal must be "at all times restrained, and kept securely confined within a totally enclosed part of the vessel from which it cannot escape". Hence the contact situation previously envisaged should no longer arise. Additionally "native" animals are banned from boarding vessels with foreign animals aboard.

At Hull in August 1977 the captain of a West German cargo ship was fined £400 and his bosun and watchman £300 each for allowing a dog on deck.

A new amendment to the Import Control Order in September 1977 barred native British animals from vessels carrying animals from abroad, and defined more precisely the security arrangements under which foreign animals must be confined on board vessels in British ports, and also designated more clearly the persons to be held responsible for such animals' confinement. The powers of the Diseases of Animals Inspectors, and the police were extended, to enable them to seize animals which are illegally landed or allowed to wander loose on deck of a vessel where it might constitute a danger. The power to have such an animal slaughtered was also given.

Local authorities, who are the enforcing authorities under the Import Control Order, already have the power to destroy animals landed illegally. Although it would seem a massive deterrent to make it mandatory that all illegally imported animals are destroyed at once, it would not be advisable for many reasons. In some cases it makes better sense to keep an animal under veterinary observation; and in cases where the offence of illegal landing was on a technicality only, such as some miswording in the import licence, it would not be fair to destroy the animal. The inference that it was the animal which would suffer would also stop many kind-hearted members of the public from lodging information about illegally landed animals, and it is to the co-operation of such people that the Ministry must inevitably look, as our coast line and harbours cannot be watched all the time everywhere. It is interesting to note that during 1975 nearly one-third of the people prosecuted for illegally landing animals chose to have them destroyed rather than to bear the costs of quarantine or of re-export to the place from which they were brought. It would seem that people are willing to take a gamble in smuggling their pets in, but if they lose, they are willing to accept that the pet must die, so mandatory destruction would not be a great additional deterrent. It is something which the smugglers have already taken into consideration.

The most extreme suggestion which has been put forward is that if it were possible to ban the entry of all rabies susceptible animals from Britain, we should be safe from the disease. Such a ban would seriously impede medical research, which imports some 40,000 animals for this purpose each year. Zoos, safari parks and also the pedigree dog and cat lovers would suffer unduly, and it would be hard to justify such a ban, when our quarantine arrangements are working so well, except for the selfish few who choose to disregard them, or think that their animals must be excepted. There is also every likelihood that if a total ban was put on the importation of dogs and cats, there would be a significant increase in illegal landings, and there might be an organised traffic in dogs and cats as contraband. The country would then be at greater risk of the introduction of rabies than it is now with a system of tightly controlled imports. Malta has recently banned completely the importation of dogs and cats from UK, as a means of controlling the embarkation of animals from boats and yachts. On such a small island, this is bound to have a deleterious effect quite soon on the quality of the island's pedigree stock.

It has been suggested that mandatory minimum penalties should be published for smuggling offences, but the Home Secretary did not agree that this would be acceptable, as the courts should maintain unfettered freedom to weigh each case according to its merits, and impose the fines and penalties which are appropriate. Fines for illegal landings have been increasing rapidly and magistrates are now applying fines closer to the maximum within their powers. The National Yacht Harbour Association, which represents most of the marina and yacht harbour operators in UK, has proposed a six point scheme which it feels would strengthen existing regulations to keep rabies out, especially in the small ports around our coasts which seem so vulnerable and about which questions are frequently asked in Parliament. In September 1976, a veterinary surgeon, writing to the Veterinary Record, complained that in bad weather it was quite common for 20 to 30 Breton fishing boats to lie up in the habour at Milford Haven, and many of these boats carried dogs and cats. Local British animals, as is the habit in country places, wander about all day, and have every opportunity to intermingle with the animals from the Breton boats. The writer said that there were no notices easily visible which could be clearly read from the quay side about the rabies situation and the control procedure. Local people were well educated about rabies, except that they did not see why they should take the trouble to keep the animals within bounds, but it seemed that there was no clear statement for the personnel of foreign ships to read. The following week a veterinary surgeon from near Littlehampton replied that it was necessary for people in the know to pester their District Councils to see that all control measures and due notification was made, and that this had been done in his area on the Sussex coast, but there was just one loophole to making the control 100% effective. MAFF had set up a control system to operate once the disease of rabies is in a town or country area, but had no powers to board a vessel to remove an animal which may be a rabies carrier. Under the amended order, however, an inspector or a constable may now board a vessel in harbour to seize an animal which is not properly confined or which may have had contact with a native animal. Anyone seeing a dog or cat leave a foreign vessel should telephone the police or the consumer protection or trading standards office to reach the right people to deal with a situation which falls between several authorities, but now powers of seizure are given to the police this will probably cover all contingencies.

Dogs and cats legally imported and arriving fully documented in their owners' cars on ferries will be met by the authorised carrying agent who will bring with him a crate of sufficient size in which to put the animal to take it to his van and the quarantine station. Where the presence of an animal is not declared or discovered until it and the owners are on board plane or ferry heading for Britain, considerable difficulties arise, for it is not very easy to find a quarantine kennel which has the space to take unexpected animals, or licensed carriers to convey them at short notice. It is also understandable that quarantine kennels are not eager to accept animals for which the owners have not made pre-bookings, for these animals may not be claimed at the end of their stay, if the owners think better of their impulse, and their bills may not be paid. At some ports, owners are offered telephone facilities by which they may make arrangements for quarantine, during which time the animal should be housed in security accommodation at the port or airport. If the animal is loose in a car, it may be that the car and animal must remain on the ferry and go back and forth across the channel until arrangements are made about the quarantine of the animal, or the owner takes the decision to have it destroyed. Destruction of the animal in no way removes from the owner the liability for prosecution for breaking importation regulations.

Imported animals cannot be sent on to distant quarantine kennels by rail. If the journey is very long, or through some mishap or failure to make prior arrangements, the hour of departure is very late, the licensed carrier may have to make an overnight stop, but this must only be with permission of MAFF, and must be at a licensed quarantine kennels on route for the final destination.

There should be no excuse for foreign visitors, or returning nationals not knowing that they cannot have their dogs with them while in Britain, unless they have been through quarantine. MAFF has issued posters in eight languages, each one treated slightly differently to fit the manners and customs of each country where it is to be displayed. For France, where rabies is widespread, the appeal is to keep rabies out of Britain.

As it is difficult to ensure that even the most strikingly designed posters are seen by everyone, amid the bustle of travel, MAFF provided in 1977 large free standing all-weather notices for ports, stating in multi languages on 2 x 3 ft boards that no animals may be landed (except by proper arrangement). Notices double the size, 6 x 4 ft mounted permanently in concrete blocks, will appear at all the main ports of entry, giving a pictorial message: an animal in a red circle, scored out by a cross. This will be in addition to the usual sized posters, notices in veterinary surgeries, and leaflets which are handed out by embassies abroad.

For some foolish people, all the posters in the world are of no use, for they have the deliberate intention of smuggling their pets into the country. By far the most usual reason for this anti-social action is an excessive affection for the pets which they are convinced will not survive separation from their owners. In fact the great majority of dogs and cats do very well in kennels and it is only the owner who finds the separation hard going. Animals are, by their very nature, adaptable, and while not being at the peak of happiness, they are able to adjust to a more boring life, provided their quarters are warm and comfortable and there is contact with friendly human beings.

The enormous increase in cross channel holiday and business traffic in the last few years, and the institution of the Green Channel at Customs, allowing people who have nothing to declare to pass through without hindrance, has undoubtedly increased the temptation to smuggle, but there is no chance that Customs will ever have the manpower to revert to individual examination of all travellers, although spot checks are always being made.

During 1975, 143 dogs and 38 cats were known to have been illegally landed, as well as 561 small mammals, many of these boxed in batches. A fair proportion of these illegal landings were technical offences only, but some were deliberate attempts at evasion. In 1976 118 dogs, 45 cats and 138 mammals were landed illegally, and there were many prosecutions, with fines ranging between £20 and £400, plus costs, and in one case, a Crown Court sentenced two offenders to three months imprisonment for deliberate smuggling and also fined them £1,000. The courts are taking a much more serious view of smuggling offences and in December 1976 a fine of £1,000 was imposed on an American lady, owner of a Maltese terrier called Muff, said to be not so much a dog, more one of the family, and positively unsuitable to endure incarceration in a kennel. Muff did do his six months in a quarantine kennel and came out looking none the worse. In addition to the £1,000 fine his owner paid £300 costs, with the threat of six months imprisonment in default of payment, all in addition to something like £250 for quarantine costs, so that smuggling attempt was dearly paid for. Muff's owner was said to be "obsessed with the dog and devoted to it". It is behaviour of this kind which makes people think mandatory destruction of every smuggled animal would work as a major deterrent – the owner of Muff would surely not have risked losing him? There are, however, many reasons against employing the destruction rule in every case, not least the time the cases take to come to trial. Muff's quarantine sojourn was over the day after his owner was sentenced. While understanding that putting a pet into quarantine for six months may be a time for great sadness and feelings of deprivation at being without a companion, it is such a selfish indulgence to put fellow humans and all *their* pets at risk. Muff the immaculate, who was, in the eyes of his owner, not as other dogs are, had been vaccinated against rabies, but this is not a total guarantee of safety and there can be no exceptions to the quarantine regime, not even for those in diplomatic circles who are normally allowed some degree of leniency in the application of our laws. Muff was, in fact, quite a danger, as he came in from Holland at a time when mass vaccination of all dogs had just been ordered, because 19 cases of rabies had been confirmed in foxes in the first two months of 1976.

Britain and the British have a longstanding tradition of pitting their wits against the Excise men, and to many people smuggling has an aura of audacity and daring which separates it from other crimes. It has always been so; in Sussex, where the low-lying coast is so suitable for illicit boating, in the 18th century nearly every class of person participated in contraband traffic and did very well out of it. The parson, preaching on Sunday to the squire, the farmer, the tradespeople and the fishermen on the sinfulness of sin and the threat of damnation to come was, as like as not, just as interested as the rest of his flock in giving shelter to a few barrels of spirits, or bales of tea and tobacco. More than once a little lost Downland church gave sanctuary to a bulky bundle or two until the dark night came around when it was safe to move the cargo on. The horses of the better off hauled the booty away, their servants providing the manpower. Smuggling was a great class unifier, and smuggling was not wicked, in the eyes of the common man; it was a fair retribution against taxes and laws imposed by those in government, who probably wanted the proceeds for their own ends. The spirit survives in many travellers who consider it fair game to bring extra spirits in beyond their duty free allowance, or another watch strapped to their thigh, another bottle of perfume deep in the brief case. Exceeding the duty free allowance does not rank very high in the list of sins to the man in the street. Smuggling provides tension and excitement, and livens up the boredom of the journey. A lot of people are guilty, and doubtless the Customs and Excise men realise it, allowing our worthy citizens their small scale fiddles to provide them a bit of fun. When you are safely in Britain, your illegal bottle is no danger to you and is easily disposed of and your conscience soon wiped clear, but even the smallest animal smuggled in is a big fiddle, a major crime in the eyes of the law and your fellow men, for it could bring rabies to Britain and death to someone close to you.

People, quite rightly, fear rabies desperately, so no one has any sympathy for the animal smuggler. There is no admiration for the clever dodge the smuggler pulled off, the way they concealed the animal and bluffed their way through. It is a story which can never be told, never as long as the smuggled animal is alive. People fear rabies more than they value family ties and loyalty, and reports have been made to the MAFF of illegal landings which must have come from close relatives of the smuggler. People always split on those who put their country in danger, even years after the deed was done. When their own lives, and those of their children are in danger, people do not hesitate to inform authority, and such information is always received and investigated in greatest confidence, for MAFF realises that the "eye of the common man" is the greatest possible safeguard against the illegal importer. Incidents of smuggled animals have been reported in the last two years which, in fact, happened several years ago. The animals must now be proved rabies free, so no action has been taken in these old cases, but it is interesting to see how the rabies awareness campaign leads people to bring up from the backs of their minds incidents which at one time they were prepared to tolerate and help conceal. People who have got their smuggled pet through customs are only just beginning on a frightening life of deception. Their continuing punishment lies in having to keep up the story of the acquisition of their pet for years and years. Dog fanciers and vets can be voluble people; in pubs and on the streets, they approach a nice friendly dog and immediately they want to know all about it, what is its pedigree, where did you buy it, and if the owner admits to coming from abroad, they will want to know how it got on in quarantine, did you go to see it, what kennel was used, only they would like to know because their Auntie wants to bring a dog in. The questions are aimiable enough, but searching because of the degree of interest, and only offensive if the dog owner cannot supply the answers without incriminating himself.

Pets constitute a basis on which strangers may converse without barriers or restraint. The burden of concealing a smuggled dog or cat, not only for the journey but for the rest of its life, may be heavy indeed. The relief when the animal, which was too dear to put in quarantine, finally dies must be very great, for only then does the threat of discovery cease. Smuggling animals seems to be largely an individual enterprise, concerned with the pets of the one owner, but there is some evidence that

Sussex still seeks to beat the Excise men, though with great reservations for this special type of cargo. John Hillaby, in his book *Journey Through Love*, published in 1976 says: "All Sussex has been implicated in the smuggling business, and at certain places they are still at it, despite what the Customs men say, but at Alfriston, the first village you come to on the Cuckmere, smuggling may be said to have been the staple industry - at the turn of the century, there was a brisk demand for eau de cologne, German cigars and naughty Tauchnitz novels. Nowadays, drugs are smuggled in concealed compartments built into cars and caravans. In Sussex the Coastal Protection Service plain clothes men are constantly on the lookout for pathetic cargoes of illegal immigrants, usually Pakistanis and Afro-Indians. And dogs, too. A lucrative if hazardous trade. Yachtsmen charge about £200 for defying quarantine regulations by landing someone's pet but they run the risk of massive fines and losing their boats if caught. The man who told me something about landing anaesthetized dogs considered it safer to ship contraceptives to Ireland."

The legend of muffled lights on cloudy nights dies hard all along the southern coasts of England, but in those counties nearest to Europe and the Channel Ports, opportunity and tradition survive. The romantic notions of "four and twenty ponies trotting through the dark" will be too expensive for the citizens of the neat little south coast resorts, if the tranquillised animal breaks away from its carriers and runs away into the forests which lie so conveniently near the coasts in these parts, to infect our pets and our wildlife with rabies, changing our way of life and the way we can enjoy our glorious South Downs scenery for a very long time. Britain will have no tolerance for animal smugglers, whether they are motivated by greed, or by affection for their pets, for with extraordinary unanimity, we mean to Keep Rabies Out.

When, in the summer of 1976, a little dog was found dead in the street in suspicious circumstances, which might be construed as rabies symptoms, holiday bookings in surprising numbers were cancelled at the town's boarding houses and hotels. The dog did not have rabies, it had probably taken some poison, but the case did show what will happen if a rabies case is diagnosed; it might rebound on the livelihood of the very fishermen who are said to be helping owners to land pets illegally.

What kind of people will attempt to smuggle animals into Britain? In an attempt to find out more about the situation and motivation of smuggling a survey was carried out on the 110 illegal landings at Kent ports which were detected in 1973. The survey emphasises the serious nature of the problem at that time and the considerable difficulties experienced by the port authorities. Movements of people and their pets between the continent and Great Britain is increasing, and removal of the traditional barriers by EEC countries was said to create a mistaken impression that the UK quarantine barrier had also been removed. As rabies spreads across Europe and becomes something which the people there must live with, they appear incredulous that Britain is free of rabies and means to remain so. In 1973, the illegal importation of dogs, cats and other pet mammals was a major problem in Kent; this was before the start of the intensive publicity campaign against illegal landings. The Kent coast is the nearest and busiest jumping off ground for visits to Europe; there are frequent ferry and hovercraft services from Boulogne, Calais, Dunkirk, Ostend and Zeebrugge to the east Kent ports of Dover, Folkestone and Pegwell Bay. The north Kent ports, Chatham, Gravesend, Isle of Grain and Sheerness, receive coasters, oil tankers and ocean going cargo vessels. The smaller resorts like Margate, Ramsgate and Sandwich have marinas for the thousands of private yachts which travel regularly to Britain and the continent, and in addition there are airports at Manston, and Ashford. The survey was made by Mr R. D. Locke, veterinary surgeon and Deputy RVO MAFF for the Eastern Region.

Because of the high traffic flow and the need to have a rapid turn round of ferries, the Green Lane customs clearance for those with nothing to declare is in operation at Dover, Folkestone and Pegwell Bay. Ferries and ships arriving at Kent ports total 10,000 in the winter months of January and February, and rise to over 25,000 each month in high summer. It would be a prodigious task to insist that customs officers inspected every passenger, car and piece of luggage; if they did the delays would be intolerable, but there was obvious need to put a stop to the amount of illegal landings of animals which were taking place. In 1972, 28 animals were landed in contravention of the law. Of this number, eight owners admitted to the ship's purser that they had animals illegally on board, and were given the option of putting the animals into quarantine or having them destroyed. Four more animals were declared to customs on arrival, customs officers detected 11 other animals, and five got through the port controls but were detected inland. During the investigation of these landings it became apparent that there was need for improvement in the lines of communication between HM Customs, local authorities and MAFF at all levels, so Mr Locke decided to obtain detailed information about every illegal landing in 1973, with the co-operation of all the other authorities in supplying the fullest possible details. At the end of 1973 information was available on 110 incidents.

As it is with the present Rabies (Importation of Dogs, Cats and Other Mammals) Order 1974, the official interpretation of the Rabies (Importation of Mammals) Order 1971, which was in operation at the time of the survey, was that an animal has landed in Britain, when it, or the vehicle which carries it, touches land. The animal is therefore considered to have landed illegally and an offence committed *before* arriving at a Customs control point. In making the survey, Mr Locke was interested not only in illegal landings, as defined above, but in potential illegal landings, when an animal embarked at a continental port without an import licence; this was considered a potential illegal landing until the owner admitted to the purser or the crew that his animal was on board ship, and it was taken back without being allowed to land; this happened in six cases. While the ferry was disembarking passengers in a British port the animal would be kept in conditions of maximum security on the ferry or ship.

The illegal landings in Kent in 1973 were sub-divided into three main groups; Group A, 10 animals which evaded port controls and were detected inland. Group B, action by the authorities which prevented 33 animals entering the country. These include those detected on board ship but not voluntarily declared; those detected by customs in the red lane, again not declared by owners, and all animals detected by customs after their owners had entered the green (nothing to declare) channel. These two groups, comprising 43 animals, obviously include the attempts to smuggle. The remaining 67 animals, where the owner had taken action, were those where the owner had declared their presence to the shipping company before embarkation, to the purser on board ship, or to the customs in the red lane. These owners usually claim that they are unaware of the regulations, including the need to have an import licence before landing.

In these illegal landings, dogs predominated, with cats next, and a surprising number of hamsters were brought in by servicemen from Germany. In their case, there was no attempt at concealment but it was said they were not sufficiently well informed of the quarantine regulations applying to small mammals. Hamsters are very rabies-susceptible, and servicemen have since been informed that it is not very suitable to bring hamsters back as pets or presents for family, for very few quarantine stations have facilities for small mammals of this type. The options open are to have the hamsters destroyed by a veterinary surgeon before landing, or to send them back to Europe by the transport by which they came. As the life of a hamster is comparatively short, it would seem invidious to go to the expense of putting them through quarantine even if accommodation was available.

Calais/Dover seems to be the favourite smugglers route, with Ostend and Zeebrugge the next most used ports of embarkation. People intent on smuggling animals are likely to travel by private car or caravan on ferries, or on the hovercraft, or in private yachts. Coaches and trains do not offer good conditions for smugglers; there are too many other people around with nothing to do but watch the actions of their fellow travellers. Lorries and their drivers are a potential and ever increasing risk owing to the huge increase in freight traffic on cross channel ferries. In the survey conducted there was no evidence that illegal landings at Kent ports were more frequent at any time of day or night, or on any day of the week, but the volume of holiday traffic in August made the detection of smuggled animals more difficult. Modern veterinary tranquillisers are very effective, and will keep animals totally quiet and inactive when there is need to secrete them, but one of the snags to their use is that the individual tolerance rate is extremely variable, even in the same breed and weight of animal. Some would-be smugglers have tranquillised their animals so successfully that they never woke up again. Other animals have been given sea-sickness tranquillisers meant for humans which on occasion have the reverse effect, making the animal agitated and uncontrollable. Cats have been given aspirin to make them sleepy, the owners being unaware that aspirin is a deadly poison to cats. Would-be smugglers usually try out the tranquillisers in a dummy run first, and some may well be deterred by the effect the drugs have on the animals. Smuggling attempts are usually pretty amateurish, efforts at concealment being half-hearted, perhaps so that there may be some alibi like "we thought you saw the dog was there" if the customs apprehend the smuggler. Dogs are covered by coats and luggage on the back seat of the car; they are put under the front seat, under blankets on the floor by the driver; in a car boot, or wrapped in a bundle of coats between the front seats. Current fashion crazes make it simple to stick a little dog under a flowing poncho, but customs men will be on the look out for the lady who feels the cold so badly on a scorching August day. Cats have arrived concealed in coloured plastic bags, or lying sedated on the car floor with luggage carefully arranged to overhang their hideyhole, or they may rest on the passenger's lap, with a cardigan just artfully draped to cover a furry bundle. A rather more devious idea was demonstrated by the lady, apparently heavily pregnant, who turned out to have a large tabby cat strapped to her stomach. It must have been un-nerving for anyone who bumped into her to hear the bulge say "miaow".

Caravans seem to offer great opportunity and temptation to smugglers but, really, it has all been thought of before. Ideas put into practice have included putting dogs inside the box seats of caravans, building special compartments in false floors of wardrobes and toilet compartments, and fixing false panels to doors where a small animal can be concealed. When customs officers make their spot checks on vehicles and passengers, they are, of course, looking for other things as well as animals, and false compartments may well conceal more valuable contraband in the odd corners of the curved caravan shape which are often covered over. The size of the dog involved does not seem a limiting factor to the smuggler – three of the dogs discovered in hiding places were Alsatians. Two rabbits were in a box under clothing, and a guinea pig was in a box hidden under other luggage. These last were probably brought in illegally in an attempt to placate children at loosing their pets, but it is never too soon to educate them on the necessity to keep rabies out.

The 10 smugglers which were apprehended inland in 1973 represent a variety of attempts to "get away with it" which failed, mainly due to information given by the general public. A French holiday maker who had travelled on the hovercraft was seen by an off-duty customs officer to stop the car outside Dover and take a cocker spaniel out of the boot. Another cocker spaniel was reported by a veterinary surgeon in Lancashire, belonging to a British girl who worked abroad; this dog had been brought in on the Hovercraft too. A British girl who had been on holiday in Corfu brought a cat back with her; neighbours at her Lancashire home tipped off the police, this cat also having come in on the Hovercraft. A

Dutch nurse arrived with a large mongrel dog in Durham; neighbours thought it was odd and informed the police. The nurse admitted that the dog had been sedated and concealed by luggage in her car. The dog was re-exported, and the nurse left the country soon after. Neighbours again were on the watch when an English woman married to a Dutchman arrived back from a European trip with two cats. She admitted that they had entered by Hovercraft, as had the Dutch nurse's dog; the cats were sitting on the owner's knee covered in coats as they came through customs. The woman was fined £50 and the husband £50 for aiding and abetting – these fines would now be much stronger as the limits have risen several times since 1973 when the survey was made. Another illegal import was only discovered when a Frenchman was found at Dover to have a cat in his car, on the way back to France. He admitted bringing it in eight days earlier. A rather more ingenious French woman had a cocker spaniel with her on the night train ferry from Dover to Victoria, London. She was apprehended at the station after railway staff and passengers had remarked on the fact that an obviously foreign traveller had a dog with her. Other illegal landings were involved in three kittens found on a wharf at Gravesend, put off a freighter from East Germany, and also a cat which escaped from a yacht of Belgian origin, while at Dover.

In 1977, a Spanish lorry driver arrived in London with a load of leather goods from Madrid, and a three week old puppy which he had picked up en route.

The President of the National Yacht Harbour Association has said that as regulations now stand, any foreign yachtsman may retain a dog or cat from abroad on board his craft in British coastal waters, and may occupy a mooring linked with the mainland, provided he understands that he must keep his animal confined on board. No account seems to be taken of the size of the animal or the space available for its confinement from either the practical or humanitarian point of view. The suggestion was made that at marinas and small harbours vessels below a certain tonnage, carrying rabies susceptible animals should be banned. This proposal did not find government favour due to the impossible task of setting a tonnage limit to be equated with the enormously varying sizes of rabies susceptible animals. The problem has not basically been the size of the vessel involved but the failure of some people to confine their animals properly, irrespective of the size of the vessel. The parliamentary secretary to the Ministry of Agriculture added that he saw no reason why marina operators should not direct boats with animals aboard to certain specified moorings, preferably those furthest from land, in order to reduce the possibility of illegal landings, and to make the problem of surveillance easier. Another suggestion was that vessels arriving from abroad with animals should fly the yellow quarantine flag, below the Red Ensign, in one hoist, at least until the Health Authority has authorised the owner to keep the animal on board, after which time an internationally agreed signal flag should be flown all the time the vessel is in British waters. This idea would need international agreement, and would take some time to bring into use, as amendments to the international code of signals only come into force every five years. It was also said that "flying the dog flag" might divert attention from those vessels which had animals on board but did not intend to declare them, and were deliberately not flying the flag. It would obviously be desirable to ban native animals from close contact with vessels moored at marinas and in ports, but this ban would not be easy to enforce with anything like 100% effectiveness, particularly with regard to cats.

This problem can only be tackled on a local basis; some ports have already imposed a ban under bye-law powers and privately owned marinas can make their own rules to prevent animals being in certain areas, and this is obviously a wise thing to do, to make as wide a barrier as possible between the native animal and any animals which may escape or be allowed off vessels which have been abroad, whether British or foreign owned. Hundreds of British small boats leave marinas every summer weekend, and although it is courtesy to tell the harbour master the destination intended, there is no necessity to do so, or any check that the destination is in fact the one that is truly intended. Many of these British people will want to take their dogs with them, and have until lately been in the habit of doing so, but now posters are displayed emphasising the dangers of illegal landings and reminding owners not to take animals across the Channel. Special publicity is arranged through yachting associations to warn their members that animals taken abroad, *whether they are landed or not*, are subject to import controls and quarantine on return to this country. In addition posters have been distributed through our embassies in France, Belgium, Holland, Luxembourg, Germany, Italy, Spain and Portugal to publicise our regulations to foreign yachting associations. It is realised that HM Customs can never hope to have sufficient staff to keep constant watch over every point on the coast where yachts can berth. This is admittedly an area where some degree of risk has to be tolerated, but that risk is kept under close scrutiny with the co-operation of the Royal Yachting Association, the National Yacht Harbours Association and other similar bodies. The increased public awareness and the concern being shown about illegal landings is a great safeguard.

Attention is often drawn to the off-shore oil rigs as being a danger area for the entry of rabies. In fact, life is extremely well disciplined on the rigs through necessity, and there is no evidence that oil-rigs present a loophole in the anti-rabies regulations. Animals landed from the rigs, whether or not they have come from outside territorial waters, and whether they have had contact with animals from Europe or other countries, are subject to the normal six months in quarantine. HM Customs as the relevant port authorities are well aware of the situation and appropriate enforcement measures are taken at those ports used by vessels which service oil rigs, and those airports used by the helicopters which fly personnel to and from the rigs.

It became apparent that conditions applying to animals arriving from overseas by air and needing transfer to inland flights were not entirely satisfactory. The identification of the imported animal once it has transferred from international to domestic flights has been tightened, so that there is no opportunity for an animal from a rabies indigenous country, or indeed anywhere overseas, to become mistaken for one making an inland flight, or a journey between the mainland and Ireland or the Channel Islands and the Isle of Man. Labelling procedures have been modified to ensure that there is no possible contact between an animal from overseas and one making an inland flight by the same plane. Regulations are now being formulated to agree at international level identification labels for all animals travelling by air which will denote their foreign or native status, the proper procedures for notifying destination airfields of imported arrivals, and limiting the type of vehicle which may be used to carry the imported animals from the aircraft and to their quarantined destination.

The licence to import an animal from overseas, whether by air or other means, should be applied for at least six weeks, and certainly not less than three weeks, before the importation date, in order that the quarantine accommodation may be booked, and the Ministry may verify that this has been done. Then there is time to issue the import licence to the carrying agent, and a "boarding document" and a red rabies control label sent to the owner or his agent overseas, which will confirm the licence number issued and also act as written evidence which a shipper or airline will require to see before allowing the animal to be embarked for this country. In addition the boarding document will give description of the animal, its colour and distinctive marks, and state that it may only be

moved from ....
(place of landing), to be taken by the nearest available route to quarantine

premises at ....
The document is signed by an officer of MAFF. All expenses in connection with the landing, transit, quarantine and vaccination are for settlement by the owner of the animal, or the person having charge of it, and neither MAFF or DAFS has responsibility for expenses or the loss, death or illness of any imported animal while in transit or in quarantine.

It is important to understand that British quarantine regulations apply to animals from all countries, excepting those off-shore previously mentioned, and not only to countries where rabies is indigenous. Thus, animals from Australia and New Zealand are subject to full quarantine in Britain, although those countries share our fortunate status in being rabies free. Dogs and cats going from Britain to Australia do not need anti-rabies vaccination, but they must have been resident in UK for the previous 12 months. This means that if an Australian breeder wished to import stock say from USA, it must come to Britain first and wait here a year. On arrival in Australia dogs and cats which have travelled by air must do 90 days quarantine, if they have not been unloaded from the aircraft during the journey. Those animals which have been unloaded, and those which have travelled by a ship which has called at intermediate ports on the journey, must spend nine months in quarantine on arrival. If the seals on the travelling box of a dog or cat travelling by air are found to be broken since they were affixed in Britain, the animal will be refused entry. This makes the journey to Australia somewhat hard going for an animal, but serves to show how much importance Australian authorities put on keeping free of rabies. Should Britain have even one case of rabies outside quarantine, all imports of animals to Australia from UK would cease. New Zealand demands that UK should have been free of rabies for 12 months and that animals shall have received two doses of Rabiffa vaccine before leaving UK. There is a considerable volume of export trade done in pedigree dogs, in which Britain is acknowledged to lead the world, but most of this would come to a stop if rabies were present in this country. British dogs enter most countries without undergoing quarantine.

Many countries will let in dogs and cats without the need to undergo quarantine if they have been resident in Britain for six months - this being an international passport to being free of rabies. Among countries making this concession are Belgium, Finland, Hawaii, Hong Kong, Trinidad and Tobago, Sweden, Malawi, and Malaysia. France requires that UK shall have been free of rabies for three years, if the animals are not vaccinated. Other countries need a certificate that no rabies exists in Britain. Argentina, Norway and Indonesia make this restriction.

Many more countries require a certificate saying that Britain has been free from rabies for the six months before the animals are exported: Barbados, Jamaica, Peru, Seychelles and Yugoslavia are on this list. The Bahamas, Mauritius, Libya and Mexico demand freedom from rabies in UK for 12 months, and in addition, animals going to Gibraltar must not land anywhere else en route. Among the few countries imposing quarantine restrictions on British dogs are Cyprus (believed free of rabies now), which requires six months quarantine, Fiji, 30 days, and the Netherlands, which imposes 30 days isolation on animals but in their place of residence, not at a quarantine station. Dogs and cats which will pass through Belgium and Luxembourg should not be vaccinated with anti-rabies vaccine in Britain, as these countries do not approve the inactivated brands of vaccine, using only the live vaccines which are not obtainable in Britain. Holland has recently agreed to accept animals vaccinated with the inactivated vaccine. Dogs and cats heading for Uganda must be vaccinated with the Flury strain vaccine which is also not obtainable here. America, where rabies is widespread in wildlife, without hope of ever being eradicated, requires no rabies precautions or certification.

It is evident that great reliance is placed by overseas countries on Britain remaining free of rabies, and that their attitude would alter dramatically if we did not maintain such stringent precautions to keep the disease out.

Our greatest risk is from the deliberately smuggled animal, brought to Britain either in ignorance of the quarantine regulations, or with a deliberate intent of evasion - perhaps from sentiment or as a gamble which sets the paying of quarantine fees against the chance of getting the animal in free - with a side bet on fine or imprisonment for the person in charge of the animal and destruction of the dog or cat when discovered. People who have lived in countries where rabies is widespread place enormous faith in the anti-rabies vaccination which they obtain for their dogs, but their pet animals are managed in a very different way from Britain. Very few dogs take exercise on their own, as so many British dogs seem to do, spending several hours each day unsupervised, mixing, matching and despoiling as the mood takes them. Only in USA is the stray and free-running dog as much a problem as in Britain and, there, rabies is with them forever. To some extent the German, Dutch and French owner can be forgiven for forgetting that Britain, while exhibiting a low standard of dog care, is one of the few countries free of rabies and intends to remain so, if for no other reason than that anti-rabies measures would cost the government, and eventually the tax-payer, millions of pounds which we can do without spending.

Probably everyone who attempts to smuggle in their pet does so in the almost certain belief that the dog or cat has not been out of their sight and could not possibly have been in contact with a rabid animal. This feeling that "our dog is different, beautifully kept and certainly not the conveyor of any disease" is at the root of many of the smuggling attempts. Very probably the belief is justified, but with such a deadly disease and so much at stake, it is manifestly not possible to make any distinctions. Rather more of a risk is the dog or cat in a small sailing vessel which may have been given a free run in a French port or on the coast, and may, during a scurry into the bushes, chased and bitten or been bitten by a rabid wild animal. One of the great deceivers of rabies infection is that it does not require great gaping wounds to penetrate a new host – the scratch or bite on an animal may not be at all noticeable.

Presumably a human being will always know when they have been bitten, but when the injury hardly breaks the skin it is difficult to regard it as serious. Another great danger is the devoted animal lover who encounters a whimpering puppy or frightened kitten while on holiday abroad, and in a mistaken upsurge of humanity plans to smuggle the ailing animal back to Britain and lots of tender loving care, but not to pay its way through quarantine, for which advance arrangements will not have been made, nor such an expense budgeted. Such a sentimental impulse may put the whole of the population and its pets at risk. The stray animal, particularly one that looks ill and is behaving with exaggerated friendliness, may be very close to showing the active symptoms of rabies. Such an animal is truly an unexploded bomb of disease and hearts should be hardened against touching the pathetic waif. There is, in Europe, a much greater gulf between the owned and cared for pet, and the straying animal than exists in Britain. British visitors abroad find the sight of wandering animals distressing, until they understand the reason why these animals are untouchable and unacceptable in the home. The visitor to Europe should also be on guard against touching any wild animal, particularly fox or badger, which is unnaturally tame.

The Ministry has, in the last two years, mounted a very large and expensive campaign to make sure that foreign visitors know that they cannot bring animals into Britain unless they undergo quarantine. The only exceptions are animals normally resident in Northern Ireland, Eire, the Channel Islands, and the Isle of Man, but animals arriving from overseas via those countries will still be subject to quarantine. All the quarantine regulations are laid down in the Rabies (Importation of Dogs, Cats and Other Mammals) Order 1974 No 2211 and Amendment orders. This order states that an animal shall be understood to have landed in Britain immediately it is unloaded, or taken out of, or in any other manner leaves or escapes from a vessel or aircraft. This includes an animal which has travelled in its owner's car on a ferry, and is still within the car on discovery - that is, the animal does not have to be walking about on land to have committed the offence. The person culpable and chargeable with any breach of quarantine regulations is the person in charge of the animal at the time, not necessarily the owner of the animal. Failure to make arrangements in advance for quarantine facilities constitutes an offence against the law, but if the presence of the animal is declared voluntarily to the captain of ship or plane, when the animal carrier becomes aware of the breach of regulations, the offence will probably be less severely regarded than if deception and concealment is maintained.

Many more pedigreed dogs were smuggled than mongrel ones, but in cats the reverse is true: four moggies were stuffed into zipped up bags for every Siamese or Persian cat that suffered the indignity. In size, as is predictable, dogs under 20 lbs in weight were the easiest to try to conceal, but in the Kent survey, 15 of the concealed dogs were between 20 and 50 lbs in weight, which is quite a lot of dog to hide, and 16 were real giants over 60 lbs in weight. These dogs must have been heavily sedated for it would take a remarkable animal indeed to lie passive without wanting to look out of the windows of car and van when it was passing through docks or customs. Big dogs especially of the guarding breeds are essentially curious and they would not normally sleep in a situation of excitement. Many of the dogs which people tried to bring in were puppies under one year old, some quite young, which people had bought or picked up as strays while they were on holiday abroad. Either they had not been warned when buying of the need to quarantine their new acquisition - or so they said; or they had received false information. Several people claimed that French or German veterinary surgeons had told them that once vaccinated the dog or cat could freely enter Britain. Others were told that all formalities about quarantine would be attended to for them once they had entered Britain. If this was so it points to a lack of communication which should now be greatly improved as senior veterinary officers from MAFF have visited their counterparts on the European coast and through them have contacted veterinary surgeons in practice all over the continent. It is difficult to believe that veterinary surgeons would give such false advice, for many European vets attend the veterinary congresses in Britain, nearly all of them speaking very good English, and veterinary surgeons from Holland, France and Germany have given papers on rabies at these conferences, informing British vets on how the disease is managed in their countries. It would seem that people quite frequently credit vets with saying what they want to hear or they do not make it clear that they are taking the dog or cat back to Britain at once. Truthfulness is not a marked attribute of the would-be smugglers. Seventy-six said they were not aware of quarantine regulations before they started the journey. One woman who made this statement, she was travelling as a passenger in the cab of a lorry, was caught attempting to smuggle a cat but she had with her a dog for which she held a correctly processed import licence. It would appear that she thought paying for quarantine for one was enough and that she would take a chance on the cat - but for her it did not work out. It is true that the dog is most associated with the quarantine laws, cats rather less so in the public mind, and few people have realised that hamsters gerbils, rabbits and mice are also subject to quarantine, and are therefore rather unsuitable to bring to UK. Only one third of the errant owners coming in through Kent ports in 1973 had enquired about the procedure for bringing in animals.

In the 110 cases, most of the dogs came originally from UK and most of the owners were British, returning to take up permanent residence in the country or British people living overseas coming back to visit relatives. But even more were British residents who had been on holiday abroad and had taken the dog with them and sought to bring it back again without quarantine. Foreign visitors were sometimes accompanied by animals, especially when making a short visit to Britain during a more extensive journey. Had they bothered to enquire, it is possible to put their animals into quarantine kennels for a short time usually a minimum of a month, provided an import licence has been obtained and prior arrangements made. When the animal is reclaimed it must be taken by licensed carrier straight to ship or plane for re-export if its period in quarantine has been shorter than six months.

Of the nationalities other than British, French, American, Italian and Dutch nationals were involved and the Hovercraft route was most often used, this being the shortest journey time lasting only 30 minutes, and the smugglers probably thought that they stood a better chance of keeping the animals concealed and sedated for this length of time. Foreign nationals showed little appreciation of the universal British feeling against those who smuggle animals in - some animals were released from hiding places quite blatantly very soon after leaving the ports, and some were even taken into hotels in the towns. The idea persists that it is only necessary to beat the Excise men; in fact it is the whole British nation that is against the person who risks bringing rabies to Britain.

Seventy of the owners in the Kent survey were listed as men, but it is believed that fathers of families took responsibility when the actual pet owner was another member of the family. When the pets were owned and brought by women, it was the unmarried younger set, aged between

21 and 35 who were most criminally inclined, followed by unmarried women aged up to 50. The younger group also claimed most frequently that they did not know the regulations, and into this age group fall the returning servicemen, who did know about dogs and cats going into quarantine but were not aware that hamsters were also covered by the regulations. Older people were not often involved in secretly bringing in pets. Not everyone could claim that they were totally devoted and committed to the animal for which they risked so much; some had owned the dog or cat for as little as 12 hours or two days, these being the strays that were "rescued" while on holiday. Other pets were more members of the family, having been owned for two years or more by people living abroad, but oddly enough, over one third of the detected smugglers elected to have the pets put down immediately rather than to try to make quarantine arrangements for them. A good number did accept the offer of the use of the police office and telephone to try to contact a quarantine kennel which would take their animal which, in the meantime, remained in the kennels of the ferry and sailed back and forth across the Channel until an official carrier could arrive to meet it, and 19 dogs and six cats were re-exported on the ferry to the country from which they came, where arrangements with relatives or friends could be made to take them. Animal smuggling cuts across all class barriers: doctors, dentists and diplomats have been involved, as well as all ranks of servicemen from private to brigadier. After the 1914/18 war, and to some extent in 1945, a blind eye was turned to the pets of returning soldiers and airmen, but in the face of the present danger, there is no room for such leniency. The outbreak of rabies in 1919/22 is thought to be directly attributable to the dogs brought back by returning soldiers. Animals are not now allowed to be brought back by any means of service transport, if any other way is available, and servicemen have made large sacrifices in the cause of keeping rabies out. The French navy does not allow any pets on board ships which are visiting British ports, and the Merchant Navy, once so dependant on the company of animals on long voyages, has banned all dogs, cats and small pets from its ships, thus depriving personnel of one of the amenities which they most valued, in the interests of national safety. In 1977, dogs were banned by the Admiralty from Royal Navy ships, so killing a tradition of ship's dog dating back to Nelson's time.

In the 1973 account, many of the smuggling attempts detected inland were made by foreign nationals, but it must be remembered that these people are more easily identified as illegally being in possession of an animal; probably an equal or larger number of British residents escaped detection for they were not noticeable once they got on land. British nationals taking their dogs out on holiday stood a better chance of escaping detection in 1973, but now that rabies awareness is the watchword, all eyes are on the car with GB plates and an animal lying on the rear parcel shelf, or the British couple exercising a dog on a sunny Spanish beach. These people are not often challenged while they are abroad, but their car numbers are taken and notified to Customs; sometimes their precise date of return is found out in conversation so that Customs are alerted to watch for them on the actual weekend of their return. It can be hardly any pleasure at all to have an animal on holiday with you which must be sedated and hidden all the time, for fear that some of your fellow countrymen may see you and arrange the wrong kind of welcoming committee. Cars with foreign number plates are equally well observed in Britain; local radio stations along the Sussex and Hampshire coast frequently broadcast messages for people to look out for cars thought to be carrying animals. Nearly always the dog is one belonging to relatives and friends being visited, but it pays to act on any slight suspicion, and the true animal lover will not bear resentment when the aim is to preserve the welfare of all pets in Britain. Police constables patrolling in south coast resorts say that throughout the hot summer of 1976 they were asked almost every day to investigate beach parties of foreign nationals who were playing with dogs – and talking to them in French, no less! Nearly always it turned out that it was the landlady's dog, or the employer's which was being given an outing and a chance to learn a bit of foreign obedience training, but the police had no objection to making gentle enquiries in a cautious and polite manner, for a potentially rabid dog on a crowded beach could be dynamite.

The huge crowds of French, Dutch and Belgian shoppers who have made shopping trips to Britain must be doing our anti-rabies campaign a lot of good, for they are afforded the opportunity to see our posters and the notices about quarantine regulations which should stick in their minds if they consider coming over for a longer stay. We hope, and the Ministry believes, that the posters are in obvious places where they cannot be missed, but an investigator from an animal charity made a test run which was illuminating. The customs shed at Calais through which both car and foot passengers pass before embarking on the ferry contained four small posters so placed that they were easily obscurred by customs personnel or passing vehicles. The boat on which the investigator travelled was well serviced with notices; this probably results in animals being declared to the officers at that time. Another channel crossing undertaken was from Zeebrugge to Britain, where no poster at all could be found, although the investigator looked carefully for them. Even more disturbing was that fact that the lady was allowed to walk right through the Green Channel of customs carrying an obvious and conventional cat basket – empty, of course. In mitigation, it may be said that the investigator in question was young, beautiful and dressed in trendy fashion, the sort of lady who might well carry her powder compact in a cat basket as the latest ethnic style, but all the same, there was the opportunity there for a bit of successful smuggling, and no one, fellow passengers or customs official, challenged her. It follows that anti-smuggling campaigns must be intensified, and natural reticence abandoned in favour of prevention methods, for the safety of all of us is at stake.

It would seem very obvious that our situation, with the threat of rabies very close to us, would be greatly improved if we had no free exercising or semi-stray dogs to act as uncontrolled spreaders of disease, especially as these animals may make contact with rabid animals of which their owners are quite ignorant, since the dogs are unsupervised for many hours of the day. The greatest danger of all, in terms of human risk, is the "latch key" dog, which roams all day but goes back to its home at night, to be received into the family situation, played with by children, when no one has any idea what the dog's contacts have been, or even if its behaviour has been normal all day. We do not have many permanently free living dogs, although there have been reports of packs of dogs living and breeding on two areas of common land in the London area, but from personal observation, it is rare to see more than two dogs running together on the streets. It is far more common to see dogs wandering around for several hours, within a few hundred yards, or even nearer to their own homes, but these are technically "stray" dogs, as they are not under control, and in a rabies outbreak situation, they are just as dangerous as the dog which has no home to go to or the dog roaming miles from home. The dog which is virtually safe from rabies is the one which is supervised, or shut into the house, all the hours of the day and night, but this kind of dog keeping is sometimes more trouble than many dog owners wish to take. If rabies does come here, many of the more casually owned dogs and cats would be destroyed at the request of their owners, or because they were not claimed within three days of being rounded up as strays. It would be a salutary lesson in better pet keeping, which some people will need to experience before they realise that one man's loose pet is another man's danger. In the event of rabies being introduced here, out attitude to pet animals and wildlife must inevitably change.

In the autumn of 1977 the Joint Animal Committee, made up of representatives of the animal charities, the veterinary associations, and local authorities, known as JACOPIS and chaired by the Rt Hon Lord Houghton of Sowerby, requested the government to institute a national dog warden service, to round up stray dogs, restore them to their owners and to help with the education of the public in good dog keeping so that their pets are not a nuisance to others. Some local authorities have already employed dog wardens, some for as little as four hours a day, but even this amount of time has shown a big improvement in the number of dogs allowed to run loose. JACOPIS feels the service should be on a national basis, paid for out of increased dog licence fees. The town of Halesowen, in the Midlands, staged a trial round-up of all loose animals on two days in February 1978. This was part of an exercise by the West Midlands Council to test its rabies contingency plans and cost around £3,500. Veterinary surgeons, police, civil servants and council officials were in attendance. When the animals were caught they were held in a multi-storey car park and owners were able to reclaim them without fee. The exercise gave encouraging proof of the ability of a county authority to carry out, quickly and effectively, its responsibility to seize and detain uncontrolled animals. It was also interesting to see that the overwhelming majority of pets were either shut up at home or kept on leads during the period of the exercise, as they would have to be in the event of a real outbreak.

Diagnosis of rabies, especially of the first case to be seen for some years, is a great responsibility to be borne by the medical and veterinary profession. It will need supreme tact to convey to a pet owner that rabies is suspected, and probably quite a lot of courage too, to set in motion all the official restrictions which will then become operative, especially if, in the end, the illness was not rabies but something more common. Ridicule and scorn may be the lot of the vet who mis-diagnoses a brain tumour as rabies; criminal negligence might be the charge if he fails to recognise the disease and through his failure the owners and children get fatally bitten.

Chapter 10

The Way It May Happen

The following account of what happened when Mrs Madge Lawrence's Cavalier King Charles Spaniel dog Toby became ill, may serve to illustrate, in everyday terms, the pattern of events which might take place should a case of rabies be diagnosed in Britain. The characters and locality are fictional; the action taken by Ministry officials, and the restrictions imposed on the area, are those which would be likely to be implemented, if a rabies outbreak occurred.

Extract from the diary of Mrs Jack Lawrence (Madge), of Rose Cottage, Foxhanger, near Beechwood, Sussex. Mrs Lawrence's husband works in the cathedral town of Westchester, 12 miles away. Also involved in the story is her sister Tina, and her husband (Alec Stack), who live near Thraxton, Surrey; and the Beechwood vet Mr Richmond and his young assistant, Rex Truman, and the Regional Veterinary Inspector of MAAF, Mr McKenzie.

February 9th.

Directly the children have gone to school tomorrow I mean to take Toby into the vet. In the last week, he has turned from being a happy bubbling little Cavalier into a old grouch, miserable, depressed and can't eat, even his companion little Lucy can't make him play. I wonder perhaps if he has toothache, as he is dribbling more and more, and he never has been a slobbery kind of dog. We had Meaty the boxer in for a few hours today while Mrs Green went out – she has shopping to do as she is taking Meaty to Crufts tomorrow – well, he may be Champion Meteor Stardust to the show world, but to us he's just a great big baby that does not like being left alone. Since the day he ripped up all the kitchen lino while she was out, I usually have him in here – my two Cavaliers don't mind him at all, they usually have a good romp with him. Lucy did today, but poor Toby was hiding under the spare room bed, and when Meaty went to look under for him, all he got was a growl for his trouble. I have never heard Toby growl before; a good thing Meaty took it like a gentleman and just walked away. Toby did come out later and ate more of his supper than he did last night, but he isn't really very interested in food, and he looks so worried – I expect it is a bad tooth.

February 10th.

Heard the Greens and Champion Meaty go off very early. They sounded excited and happy, which was more than we were; it was one of those days when everyone gets irritable. Toby wouldn't come downstairs, he was under the children's bed this time, and though they tried, and I called he wouldn't take any notice of any of us – so unlike him, he always looks for a biscuit in the mornings. My husband Jack got up a bit cross, through the Greens and their friends banging the car door and making a lot of noise about loading Meaty and all his show equipment, before 5 a.m. that was, so Jack said he was not going to stand any nonsense from *our* dog. I said to leave him be, I would get him out in time to go to the 9 a.m. surgery in Beechwood, but Jack, all red in the face, said the dog must learn who is master. Jack got down on the floor to drag Toby out from under the divan. Next thing Jack was dancing about, using all sorts of language. Toby had bitten him, Jack was dripping on the carpet, and Toby was still lying against the wall under the bed. It wasn't much of a bite, more a couple of tooth marks, but Jack was so cross, he wouldn't stop to let me put a plaster on it, but slammed out of the house and up the road to get the bus to Westchester, saying he would leave the car for me to take the *** dog into the vet's. When the children had gone and the house was quieter, I went back upstairs to see if I could coax Toby out. Well, if the little dear is feeling bad, it's no use shouting at him, but as soon as I opened the door to the children's room, Toby shot past me like a champagne cork out of a bottle, straight down the stairs out of the kitchen door and through the gate Jack had left open in his temper. The bitch, Lucy, thinking here was some fun going at last, rushed after Toby, and there they were, streaking up the lane, running faster than I have ever seen them, deaf to all my calling. I was thankful when Toby went through the hedge and across the field on to the Downs; at least they are safe from traffic there. I grabbed the leads and started after them, for I know the gamekeepers in the Forestry Commission plantation are very hot on the dogs which chase pheasants up there. By the time that I got to the Forest gate, Lucy was coming back towards me, so I put her lead on, and walked up the rides calling Toby, but there was no sign of him, and when I stood still, no movement at all in the undergrowth, so I thought he must have gone a good way already. Really, I could almost agree with Jack; the dog is getting to be a nuisance, being surly, then biting and now running off, when usually he is even more loving than Lucy. I know from past experience, it is no use walking on and on through the forest after a dog when you don't know what direction it has taken, so Lucy and I went home, and I gave up the idea of going to Beechwood – well, I almost had, when I saw Toby come crawling in at the gate. I thought at first he must have been hit by a car, he was wet, dirty and absolutely exhausted, but there were no marks on him, and he did seem quite pleased to see me and to be home; but I thought to myself, it's the vet for you, my boy. We'll just make it by the end of surgery if we hurry.

By the time we got to Beechwood, it was almost eleven, and the surgery was nearly over. I was glad the waiting room was not full, as Toby looked such a mess, like a dog nobody cared about, and as if he had not been groomed for weeks. I just nodded to Col. Transon as he went in with his rheumaticky old labrador, then there was a lady with a cat in a basket, leaving only a man with a brief case on his knees, and us in the waiting room.

Old Mr Richmond had just beckoned us into the consulting room when he noticed the man with the brief case looking hard at his watch – he had obviously been waiting for some time, a pharmaceutical company rep, I should guess. Anyway, Mr Richmond was very nice. 'Mrs Lawrence,' he said, 'I am going to leave you with my new assistant, Rex Truman, one of the bright new boys, been working in America for the last two years.' I couldn't make a fuss, as I was so late getting into surgery, but I do prefer to see Mr Richmond if I can, but this young Mr Truman seemed nice enough. He lifted Toby on to the examining table and asked me what was wrong. Toby was still very quiet, tired from all the running he had done, I expect, so it seemed a bit silly to say, 'He's different, he's not our Toby.' Mr Truman probably thought I was a silly woman, but he did not show it; he wanted to know exactly when Toby started to behave like this, if he was eating, all the details. He was interested in the drooling too, when had that started, and was it getting worse? I had to agree it had. Mr Truman opened Toby's mouth to look in and said he could not see a bad tooth, but he did give me an odd look when I said, 'Mind he does not bite you. He had Jack this morning just before he ran off into the forest.' Funny young man, instead of going on examining the dog, he suddenly said, 'Mrs Lawrence, where did you go for your holiday last year?' I told him we went to Scarborough, to Jack's people, like we always do. Then, instead of taking Toby's temperature, like they usually do, he kept walking round and round the table, looking at him from all angles, and poor Toby just stood there drooping his head, with all his lovely white fur wet and sticky. I did wish we had seen Mr Richmond, for it seemed to me that this young man did not know what to do next. Finally, he turned to me and asked if Toby had been in any fights. Well now, Cavaliers are the sweetest natured dogs, never fighters, but I did remember, because it was so unusual, Toby and my sister's Westie had such a squabble when we were at their place at Christmas – Alec, that's her husband, squirted them with the soda syphon to make them break it up. We couldn't understand them fighting, they are usually such good friends. Perhaps it was the children and all the excitement. When I groomed Toby next day I found just a little bite mark on his leg, but it wasn't really anything to worry about, so I put some ointment on it – well you can't be running to the vet all the time, can you? I told Mr Truman all that. I was beginning to feel sorry for the boy, I thought he wanted to keep me talking until Mr Richmond came back to help him out. Then, would you believe it . . . this young vet wanted to know where Alec and Tina (she's my younger sister) went for their holiday – properly obsessed with holidays this boy, perhaps he should have been a travel agent. So I said a bit sharpish, they went touring in Europe with their new car and caravan, and I had something better to do than tell him our family history, so perhaps I had better come back again when Mr Richmond was free. That seemed to do it. 'Touring', he said. 'Touring Europe . . .' He seemed to be mulling that over. Suddenly, as if he had made his mind up, he said, 'Look, Mrs Lawrence, I'm not sure about Toby, I'd like to have a colleague of mine look at him, if you don't mind.' I really felt impatient. All this time, and still can't say what poor little Toby has got, I went to pick up Toby from the table and said, sharply enough to let him know what I thought, 'I'll come back another time.' But before I could get to Toby, this young man had me by the arm, out of the door and into the waiting room, saying he must keep Toby for an hour or two, would I ring up at five o'clock, and positively hustling me out of the place, but just as I was going to the car he called out, 'Mrs Lawrence, where does your husband work?' If it hadn't been the boy looked so young and flustered, I really would have given him a piece of my mind. 'It's the dog I've come about,' I should have said. 'Why don't you find out what's wrong with him instead of keeping on about my family and my husband's work, and holidays?' I mean to say, being freindly is one thing, but all this chat when you want a professional job done. But then I thought, perhaps the lad's embarrassed, having to say he doesn't know, so I told him Jack worked at the United Bank in Westchester, and had these last 15 years, as anyone in Foxhanger could tell him, and then I came home, without Toby, and all the way I was wandering if I should have left him like that, and whether all this was going to cost a lot, and whether this young Rex Truman was really going to get another opinion, or just go and look up his textbooks. Anyway, Lucy was very glad to see me when I got back, thank goodness she seems perfectly all right, so I got on with my housework, but thinking of Toby all the time, and about Meaty too. I wondered if he was pleasing the judges up at Crufts, and if the Greens were having a good time.

I did not have long to wait. Just after 2 p.m. Mr Truman rang up to say his colleague had been to see Toby, and they both thought that whatever it was he has might be infectious, and he should be isolated for a day or two – only not at the veterinary hospital in Beechwood. This other vet would take him to his place – a Veterinary Investigation Centre, he said, more secure there. Well, as I had told him about Toby getting out that morning, I couldn't argue, but really, it did seem to be making a lot of fuss to be taking Toby miles away. And then, just as I put the phone down, in walked Jack. Jack home, and the bank not even closed! My heart turned over; was he ill, was it one of the children, it all raced through my mind. No, he said, 'It's Toby. You know what they think he's got? Rabies, that's what. Rabies. Our Toby.'

That young Rex Truman had certainly been busy since I left the veterinary hospital. He got Jack on the telephone right away, and Jack told them where Alec and Tina lived, and in another hour two policemen were there asking *them* questions, and wanting to see Timmy. If that Mr Truman had not rushed me out of the surgery, I was going to tell him that the fight with Toby must have been too much for old Timmy, for when Tina came down in the morning a few days later, he was lying dead in the kitchen. He had not seemed ill, just a bit quiet and off his food, and lame in the back legs, but then he was old and rheumaticky anyway. Alec buried him in the garden and they decided not to have another dog, not as they like to go abroad a couple of times a year. I don't know how I'll face Tina and Alec, they'll think it all my fault. These policemen wanted to know all about their holiday and whether they took Timmy with them, and if they had not had the receipt to show from the boarding kennels, where he always goes, I don't know what will happen. Tina was very sharp with me and said I was trying to get her into trouble, but as Springwood Kennels know Timmy well, the police were able to make a check there.

Jack has to go up to the doctor's tonight, to get his vaccination against rabies. They are sending some of the new vaccine down from London so that he can have it straight away, and if it turns out as bad as they think with Toby, the rest of us will have to be done too, just to be on the safe side. Thank goodness we are to have the latest vaccine, which only needs about four little injections, not those horrifying ones in the stomach we have read about. I keep wondering how could our Toby have got rabies — I look after the dogs so carefully. Jack looks dreadfully worried — he says we must not say anything to alarm the children or the neighbours, it might not be so serious after all.

February 10th.

Mrs Green wanted to come in with Meaty and tell me all about Crufts Show, but I couldn't let her in, for one thing we were told not to have any animals in the house, and then, once we got talking, I might have let it out about Toby. She looked very put out when I said I was too busy.

February 11th.

We heard today. They are pretty sure that Toby has rabies, he has been raging and biting at the cage they have him in, and when he could not get at anyone, he started tearing at his own paws. Anything more unlike our gentle Toby I can't imagine. A very nice man, Mr McKenzie from the Ministry of Agriculture, came to see us. Jack stayed home from the bank. Mr McKenzie explained that now it looks almost definite that Toby has rabies. The Ministry has a lot of power which they could, if necessary enforce by law, but he was sure we would be co-operative. He said they would have to put Toby to sleep now, so that they could examine his brain. We could not really argue, for anyway it seems that Toby is too ill ever to be our pet again, but Lucy, dear little Lucy, not her too! Lucy has to go to a Veterinary Investigation Centre, probably the same one to which they took Toby from the vet's, for 15 days, to see if she develops rabies too. We could have kept her isolated within the house but, in view of the risk to the children, Jack said she must go away. If signs of rabies show, she will have to be put down; if she is all right after 15 days, if we are willing to pay, and Jack says we will find the money somehow, she can go on to a quarantine kennel, to remain for 6 months just like a dog from abroad. I thought we would have a day or two to think it over, but as soon as the decision was made, Mr McKenzie was on the phone and a van from the Ministry came to take Lucy away. The men who came to get her wore special protective clothing, and put her into a strong cage before lifting her into the van. I thought we might have driven her in the car, but we were not allowed to. Mrs Green was in the front garden, her eyes were sticking out on stalks, she must know something is going on. I suppose we will have to tell her soon.

February 12th.

Mr McKenzie came and told us this afternoon. Toby did have rabies. He gave us a form saying that the house was an 'infected place', and put a great big notice on the gate warning people against rabies. There are posters all over the village, and on the gate into the forest. Then Mr McKenzie sat with us and went over and over the story of Timmy and Toby having the fight, and how Toby ran off the other morning, and where we have been since Christmas, and what other dogs Toby might have met. Someone else had gone to see Tina and Alec again, they think that Timmy might have died of rabies too. All the contacts have to be traced. While we were talking, Mrs Green burst in the door, almost hysterical. I was glad Mr McKenzie was here to explain to her for she was beside herself; her Champion Boxer, he was here, he was a contact, and then he went to the big show in London, hundreds of dogs were there, the cream of the British dogs – oh, how she went on! Time and time again, Mr McKenzie told her things would be all right; no, of course all the dogs would not have to be shot at once. What nonsense, he said, with any luck at all the Ministry would trace the source of the outbreak and stop it spreading and perhaps there would be no more cases at all. As for Meaty, as he is a contact to a known case of rabies, he has to go into quarantine for 6 months. I do not know if the Green's will have to pay for him or not — the alternative would be to have him destroyed, I suppose. Molly Green is heartbroken, she adores that dog, and even more the social life they get through showing him and going to dog clubs. I reminded Molly that Toby did not go very close to Meaty and certainly never bit him, so there is every chance that Meaty will be all right, and come out of quarantine quite healthy and happy. Another complication is that Meaty was at Crufts, and while there, he was in contact with any number of other dogs, in the show ring, and those benched alongside him — in fact, nearly all the best boxers in the country. All these dogs will have to be traced by the Kennel Club, and they then have to be put under 'house arrest' confined within their owners' homes for 15 days. Dear old Meaty will be examined daily, and if, after 15 days from the time he left Crufts, he is still healthy, then the restrictions on his contacts will be removed. Mr McKenzie said that the reasoning behind this is that if Meaty has not developed rabies within 15 days of Crufts, he could not have been infectious at the time he was at the show, even though there is still the possibility that he may have contracted the disease from Toby and still be incubating it. The owners of the 'contact' boxers are, of course, worried, and even more, disappointed that they cannot attend shows for two weeks; I believe the Midlands Club had a big show scheduled; I suppose that will be cancelled now as so many of the boxers are contacts and confined to their homes. Molly Green is so *silly*. I offered to make her a cup of coffee to calm her down, and she turned quite white and said she would not have anything in our house, thank you, it might be catching. It was while I was seeing her out that I noticed the first man at the gate, and then the village taxi drove up with two more — reporters from the big papers — and then a TV van turned into the lane. Mr McKenzie said not to give any interviews, but the men are still waiting.

It was on the radio news – all the country for about 15 miles around here including Foxhanger and Beechwood has been declared an Infected Area and posters and notices about it are going up all over the place. Seems like the eyes of all the country, even the world, are on our little corner of Sussex. Someone said in an interview that buyers in Australia who had bought dogs at Crufts would no longer take them, now we had rabies, and all the export trade in dogs is ruined, because of Toby. The Infected Area will take in the holiday places along the coast, well past Westchester, almost to Landport. People cannot take their dogs and cats out of this area, nor can any come in. It will be rough on people who might be staying down here, there are always a good few visitors even in winter. All the dog shows and race meetings are cancelled, the meets of the hunt and the point to point, and all the dog training classes and things like that, even the greyhound racing at Landport. Pheasant shooting is over, so that will not be affected, but no one is allowed to shoot rabbits and pigeons, so as not to scatter the wild animals who might have been in contact with Toby. Dogs can only go out if they are on the lead and wearing muzzles. It said on the radio that muzzles would be in the pet shops in about a week. They are not going to be issued free, people who want them will have to buy them; of course, a lot of people will prefer to keep their dogs indoors or in their gardens. Cats have got to be kept in their houses and people will have to arrange dirt trays for them, or else they will have to go out on leads, but I can't see any of the cats around here standing for that. All the stray dogs and cats are to be rounded up – that will be a big shock to people in the village. They don't think their dogs are strays, but they walk about most of the day as they wish, or sit outside their houses, and Mr McKenzie said that would not do anymore. When he says inside, he really means inside, not even in the garden unless the fence is high and strong so the dog cannot get over. Any dog found loose will be collected up, they are not prepared to argue about it, and of course, cats too. Men from the Westchester and surrounding local authorities are in charge of rounding up the stray dogs and cats. It really is a big job for them, as they have to be looked after and fed while they are waiting to be claimed, and the people who want to get their pets back have to be shown the dogs and made to sign forms to claim ownership and all that. It is a tremendous task, and people from the dog clubs are helping out all they can. The Sportsdrome at Wunderlins holiday camp has been taken over as a temporary home for the strays, and people can go and claim them there, but probably not to take them away just yet, until it is seen if they have rabies. The owners will have to pay all their expenses for the stay too, and the Ministry has the right to keep them as long as it seems necessary. People have to claim the animals within three days, which seems a rather short time, but Mr McKenzie says that people who want their animals normally claim them in 48 hours anyway. The dogs and cats not claimed will be put down. I can't bear to think that this is all because of Toby. The children came in crying, the other kids had been on at them at school, about losing their pets because of our dog. It seems so unfair, it's not as if we have done anything wicked. Jack is not going to work, he says he can't stand all the jokes and questions, and the way the others keep pretending to bark and that. It's bad enough to have all this worry without other people making our lives unbearable.

When Jack went for his vaccination, Dr Wilson explained to him ever so carefully that he was in hardly any danger at all, as he had the vaccine very soon after Toby bit him, and it was not a deep bite or on his head or face, which is the worst place. The children and I are going for our vaccinations tonight. Jack said it was quickly done, and his arm is only a bit sore and stiff, not really painful.

Rex Truman the vet was interviewed on TV tonight, by the President of the British Veterinary Association. They seem ever so pleased with him for finding out what Toby had, as they said it would have been very easy to miss it, and even if he thought it might be rabies, it took a bit of courage to follow his hunch, as he could have looked very silly if he had been wrong. I was wondering myself what made him think of rabies; of course, he had seen cases when he was in America, but he said it was the strange, fixed stare, the 'not with us' look in Toby's eyes which finally made him think it could be rabies and not some other brain disease.

February 13th.

We had Mr McKenzie here again today and two of his bosses, going over the story again and again, trying to help us remember something which could give them a lead. As they explained, they believe us, they don't think Toby was the first case, and it's that first case they have to find, in order to step on the outbreak really hard and save it from being in Britain for months, years, perhaps for ever. Try as we may, we can't seem to help them. They want to know if we had visitors from France or Germany who had animals with them, if we took a day trip to the French coast, if we sat near people on the beach last year who might have come off yachts with dogs, even if we let Toby run free down by the moorings at Cawley Creek, and perhaps run on to a moored yacht. But we'd never let him go out of our sight, and the fight with Timmy at Christmas was the first Toby ever had. Of course, I do take the dogs into Westchester Training Club classes and match evenings; the last one was a day or two before Toby started going peculiar. That started Mr McKenzie up again. He wanted the address of the secretary, so that he can trace all the dogs that were there. Apparently all the dogs that were at Training Club that night are to be regarded as contacts, for Mr McKenzie feels that Toby was almost certainly infectious for a day or two before he went so strange. All the dogs that were there have to be under restrictions, in quarantine for 6 months. I can hardly bear to think what the owners are saying about me; there were all sorts of dogs there, some only pets learning obedience, some show dogs polishing up their ringcraft, and then there was a kindergarten class of puppies under 6 months old learning elementary commands and how to socialise with other dogs. Some of the show dogs went to Crufts too, so all that has to be checked and the contacts in their breeds will have to be kept in house arrest for 15 days as well. I know Rosie's keeshond was there, and two of Ann's alsatians, so that is a whole lot more animals to be contacted and kept indoors. What enormous repercussions this one case of rabies is having, and try as we may, we cannot in any way account for this happening to Toby. I think Mr McKenzie believes us, but some of the other people who have asked us questions make us feel like criminals. They seem to insinuate that we know more than we will say. I thought all these dogs would have to be injected with anti-rabies vaccine, and, perhaps, all the dogs in the area, but apparently this is a decision to be made by the Ministry if the rabies outbreak warrants it.

Mr McKenzie said it would all be so easy for them if Tina's Timmy had been taken abroad with them and brought back illegally, or even if he had been through quarantine, if there had been some connection with a rabies country, but Alec and Tina can prove Timmy was in kennels all the while they were away. All the same, Tina's house in Thraxton has been declared an Infected Place, and the Ministry men dug up poor Timmy's body and took it away. Tina tried to stop them, she was crying bitterly when she told me on the phone, but it seems the Ministry have the right to take the body if they have any suspicion that an animal died of rabies, and Tina is obliged by law to tell them all she knows about Timmy's illness and death. They have been saying this on radio and TV every day –

people must tell anything they know which will be a help. Tina was very much against having 'Infected Place' on her nice house – after all, they don't even have a dog now – and she took it hard that they asked her to disinfect the house, but when they said they would get it done if she did not do it, she soon gave in. She did not want to see council cleaners going over her velvet chairs, and anyway, she would have to pay for the work, so Alec told her to get on and do it like they said.

February 14th.

Several army lorries went up the lane to the forest today. Soldiers are laying poison all over the downland and the forest to kill all the foxes in case Toby bit any while he was up there. Mr McKenzie says it is not very likely but they can't afford to take any chances. The farmers are taking their cattle and horses in, and moving the sheep to pens down near the farm just in case a rabid fox comes out of the forest. I have been doing our disinfecting, just the way Mr McKenzie told me. At least it is something to get on with, it saves me looking out of the windows, seeing people staring at the house, obviously talking about all the trouble we seem to have brought on the neighbourhood; it feels as if we have the plague. The disinfection routine is not at all bad, not a bit like being fumigated. It is really only a big springclean, with extra special washing of floors, carpets, lower parts of the walls, and any chairs the dogs sat in, with soap and household disinfectant. The beds under which Toby hid we had to turn over and go all over the springs with strong disinfectant and hot water, and they told me to wear gloves while I did it. The dogs' baskets, brushes and rugs have all been taken away by the Ministry. Jack went all over the inside of the car too, as Toby went to Beechwood in that, the very last time we saw him.

February 15th.

The Ministry men have been to Springwood Kennels where Timmy spent two weeks in September, looking at their books and getting names and addresses of all the owners of dogs and cats boarding at the same time. There must be hundreds of people working on this enquiry, they are making it more important than a murder hunt. Mr McKenzie says it is worse than murder, for who knows where the disease will strike again? Even though we are so closely involved, I have to admire the determination of the Ministry in trying to trace the original case, and also the way they are working to keep the risk of disease within this area. It seems to us that a lot of people and animals are suffering restrictions around here, but it would be far more serious if a rabies case were found in London or some other big town.

February 16th.

Mr McKenzie said that it now seems likely that in the Infected Area the local dogs and cats will receive anti-rabies injections. Probably they will book the Scout Hall for the day, and local vets will do two-hour shifts giving the injections, which will be free. Dogs, he said, almost never get any reaction to the jabs, but cats may go off their food for a day or two.

The Canine Society people are ready to help if the vaccination session is laid on; they could be a lot of use holding the dogs, making out the vaccination certificates and issuing the tags which vaccinated dogs must wear on their collars. A lot of people will have to find their dog licences and see they have an up-to-date one, if they do take their dogs to a vaccination session.

I heard that the local vets are snowed under by people who want their dogs vaccinated privately, but it is Government policy that no vaccine is being released unless MAFF considers that the general vaccination of all dogs and cats in the area is necessary.

The Canine Society people feel very resentful. Many of them have their dogs under restrictions, and even those who were not there on Toby's last night are covered by the Rabies Control Order which forbids them to take their dogs outside the area and to hold meetings in the area. Not many dogs have their muzzles yet, although a supply was rushed to the pet shops as soon as the news about Toby was known, and I understand that plastics factories are working night and day to turn out muzzles in case rabies should spread across the country. Boxers and pekes and dogs with short faces have such difficulty in getting a muzzle to fit and be effective. Last time there was a muzzling order in Britain there were no boxers in the country at all, so no one has much experience at fitting muzzles on to their funny faces, though I did hear that vets had been testing out muzzles on labs and boxers long before this awful crisis happened. The kind of muzzle which suits a labrador cuts right across the middle of a boxer's eyes, and goodness knows how it would fit a peke, even in a small size. Muzzles are not being issued free, people who want them have to buy them in the normal way at pet shops, but quite a lot of people are deciding not to take their dogs out, so they won't need muzzles. They are afraid that even if their dog is securely muzzled up, a rabid animal might rush up and inflict a bite. The newest muzzles are made of plastic, so they can be washed clean of saliva, and some are being invented that have disposable tissue linings which can be burnt. Not many people are taking dogs out even if they have enough garden to let them run in. Some dogs, like the guide dogs for the blind and the police dogs, are, by special permission, allowed to work normally. Cats are the big worry. Some people are building rabbit hutch type houses in the garden for them, as otherwise they have to stay entirely in the house.

February 17th.

The Ministry enquiries made around Thraxton seem to be bringing in some information. Several people said that their cats disappeared around Christmas time. One woman remembered a tabby cat which was cornered in a bus shelter, spitting and hissing and behaving so savagely that she wondered if it was a rare wild cat. Thraxton Common and a big area around it has been declared an Infected Area now too. At the big psychiatric hospital on the edge of the common there are masses of cats, living in the store rooms and basements; the patients and the staff feed them but they are all rather nervous and half wild. A colony of semi-domestic cats like this is a great nuisance, Mr McKenzie says. If rabies broke out among them, no one would know how many there were supposed to be, nor even where they all live. I think the hospital authorities are going to have a campaign to catch and get rid of all of the cats now – a pity because the patients used to enjoy watching them.

All the stray dogs around Thraxton are being rounded up, but no dogs are being vaccinated there yet. Alec and Tina are going for the course of anti-rabies vaccination too, just to be on the safe side. Even though it is some time since Timmy died, if by chance Alec or Tina got some of his infected saliva in a cut or a cracked finger, they could be incubating rabies. Although it is best to get treatment straight away, it is still worth having the injections two or three months afterwards, to try to get some antibodies forming in the blood. It will be a long while before any of us can feel relaxed about the chance that we may have rabies, and I expect every little headache or flu-ish cold will have us very worried. This is one of the worst aspects of the disease, not feeling safe from it for so long after you have had a contact. The vaccinations Jack and I had have left no marks, and even the children are not complaining about their arms very much. What a mercy they did not have to take the old rabies treatment with 14 or more big syringefuls to the stomach area. We all had our vaccinations on the National Health.

There are big notices posted in our forest, and on Thraxton Common to warn people that poison has been laid for the foxes – they are putting a deadly poison into chicken necks. The notice also says that all fox carcases belong to the Ministry and may only be taken away by them. The farmers are obliged to let the Ministry men and their helpers across their access land, but the Ministry do not have powers to enter gardens without the owners' permission, unless there actually is a case, or a suspect case, of rabies there. Although the poisoned bait is a great danger, at least there should be no dogs and cats loose to take it; if the Ministry people see a dog or cat they can take it into custody straight away.

February 20th.

Something happened today, something so awful it hardly bears telling. When the Ministry set about tracing all the owners of dogs which were in Springwood Kennels at the same time as Timmy they called upon them all and interviewed them. One man whose alsatian had been in the kennels said he knew Alec and Tina, he is a builder who did a bit of work on their roof early this autumn, and of course he had seen the story of Timmy and Toby in the papers. He said it was a shame about Timmy, a nice old dog; he felt sorry for him when the Stacks got that kitten, it isn't fair on an old dog to have a young thing harassing him, always on at him to play.

'Kitten?' said the Ministry man, 'The Stacks haven't got a kitten, or cat either.'

'Did have when I was working for them', said the builder. 'Straight after their holiday they had this poor little cat, vomiting, diarrhoea, it had the lot. Don't know why they bothered with it. I remember particularly because Mrs Stack asked me to keep an eye on it while she went to fetch Timmy from the kennels, and I said I had only just got my dog out – we both got back from our holiday about the same time, see – and I made the Stack's job the first on my list.'

The Ministry investigator was straight round to see Tina, and the whole story came out. The last night they were in France, they were having supper under the awning of their caravan when this poor thin little cat came mewing around. It looked half starved, and was so grateful for the bits they gave it, it curled up on the cushions and went straight to sleep. In the morning they tried to get it to go away, but it kept coming back, and Tina thought if it stayed so near the road it would be certain to get run over. As Tina said, it had adopted them; they could not be so cruel as to turn it away. Alec mentioned quarantine, but Tina would have that was only for dogs, and the long and short of it was that the cat stayed in the caravan until they drove on to the ferry. When they went down to the bar on the ship, Alec made Tina read the notice about not bringing dogs and cats or any other mammals into Britain without an import licence and quarantine arrangements being made. To give her her due, Tina was dreadfully upset when she read the notice, she saw at once she had got them in an awful fix. If they had confessed to the officers on the ferry that they had a cat with them, for which they had made no prior arrangements, they could see they would be in for a great deal of fuss and officialdom, and then there would be the considerable cost of quarantine for the cat. They did not know how much but, as Alec said, he did not feel like paying anything for a mangy little stray they did not want, and only got landed with because of Tina's impulsiveness. They sat in the car and argued for some time. Tina said she sat there with tears streaming down her face and challenged him to throw the cat overboard then, which she knew very well Alec would never dream of doing. So they decided in the end, as Alec said, to 'chance it' through the Green Channel of customs, and Tina put the cat in her knitting bag when no one was looking, and, as it happened, they got through without being challenged.

To be fair to them, I think it was true that they never thought that the cat might be the means of bringing rabies to this country, and of the danger in which they might be putting themselves, and us, and come to that, our children. It could all have been so much worse. They thought that the import licence and the quarantine regulations were just formalities that the government invents to make life difficult. They knew that dogs could not go in and out of the country, for they had always abided by that with Timmy, but Tina really thought that cats did not matter – at least, until she got on the ferry she did, and after that, well, let's say she panicked when she was faced with confessing to authority. I think Tina knew how I would feel about the rabies risk, so they did not say anything to us. They planned to let a few weeks go by and then say a stray cat had walked into the garden. From all we heard, Tina really did her best by that little cat, fed it and looked after it, even took it to the vet about its feeding problems, but the vet just told her that it had been starved most of its life and now she was overfeeding it a bit. Well, he could not possibly tell it was not a British cat, could he? One day, though, in spite of all Tina had done for it, the cat went out and did not come back, and they never saw it anymore. Ungrateful little beast, Alec said, but Timmy was glad to see the back of it. As the cat had gone before we went up there for Christmas, of course, it was never mentioned at all.

As Mr McKenzie said, the cat was probably semi-wild anyway, and already incubating rabies when Tina brought it home. When the active symptoms began to show, it must have bitten or scratched Timmy, or perhaps Timmy licked up some of its saliva, and then the cat ran off on to the common where it probably went into the furious form of the disease; cats show that form more frequently than dogs. The little cat probably ran around on the common, biting and clawing one or two other cats before it died, and we must just hope that no human touched it and got scratched. Timmy got rabies in the dumb form, with just the short time of irritability when he and Toby fought at Christmas, but quite soon after the paralysis set in, and Timmy died quietly. I suppose if he had not been so old, Tina might have consulted a vet about him when he began to be ill and get lame, but on the other hand, with her guilty secret, maybe she would not have; but no, to be honest I don't think she connected the cat or Timmy with rabies, she had never taken much interest, and if she thought at all, she pictured only dogs rushing about roaring and biting everything in sight, like mad lions. No, I think Tina really thought it was old age that killed Timmy, but we shall never know. Anyway, they buried him in the garden and thought that was the end of the story, but for us and a great many other people, the story was only just beginning.

There was all the worry to come for us, worry we still have that will be with us for a long time, because of Jack being bitten, though I must say he seems very confident of the vaccination protecting him. There is all the distress the other pet owners have had, and all the loss of wild creatures, all the fixtures for activity that have been cancelled and all the expense the country has been put to, rounding up the strays and clearing out the foxes, and vaccinating all the dogs at Westchester March meeting, all caused by Tina's impulsive kindness to a stray kitten in France.

February 27th.

It is now 15 days since the nightmare started. There have been no more cases among the dogs under 'house arrest' since Crufts, and Meaty seems well and reasonably happy in quarantine. It is so awful that there is no way to diagnose rabies until the dog or cat is dead and the laboratory can open up its brain. People like Mrs Green are in terrible suspense, wondering whether their dogs did take rabies from Toby or not. We must hope the worst is over, and there will not need to be any more slaughter of wild creatures on Thraxton Common, or in the forest here, but it will be some time before people can walk freely on those areas again, just in case some of the poisoned bait has been lifted by birds and dropped where the clearance team did not find it. Restrictions on sporting events, dog shows and so on will have to stay for some time yet, and dogs are still being kept on leads. Now people have got into the habit of keeping dogs in their gardens and under control, perhaps we shall never have quite so many dogs running loose again, to foul pavements and generally make a nuisance of themselves. A great many dogs were put down, some hundreds in the whole area, but I suppose the owners did not want them very much anyway, and took the opportunity to be rid of them without having to face up to the ordeal of taking them into the vet and asking for them to be killed. I just hope they do not take on another dog just as casually when all this trouble is forgotten, as I hope one day it will be, except for Tina and some others like her who have learned their lesson.

Our little Lucy is quite happy in quarantine, the kennel people tell us. I shall go and see her soon, but she will have to stay for the full six months as a precaution, as she was with Toby all the time. I am so glad that Mr McKenzie allowed her to go to quarantine, and that Jack was willing to pay for it; otherwise, she would have had to be put down, I think. It has been a nightmare for all of us, but all I can say is, if it had not been for young Rex Truman and his questions about holidays, and the persistence of the Ministry men in searching out the contacts that led eventually to Tina's smuggled cat, it might have been very much worse for us, and for all the people in Britain."

Chapter 11

The Deterrents

The Rabies Control Order 1974, No 2212 states:

A person who knows or suspects that an animal, in captivity or wild, is affected with rabies, or has died of rabies, must give notice of the fact to a Ministry of Agriculture, Fisheries and Food Inspector, or to a police constable.

A person who knows or suspects that an animal died of rabies must not destroy the carcase, but must keep it separately and make it available for the Ministry to see. The owner of the animal, or the occupier of the premises where the animal has been kept, and any vet who attended it, must give any information they possess and must allow facilities to the Ministry Inspector to make enquiries, to take samples, or remove the carcase. The clause in the order effectively breaks the seal of confidentiality between client and animal owner which normally appertains in veterinary surgery. A vet will, if necessary, over-rule his client's wishes, to report a suspected case of rabies.

When the Ministry Inspector has reason to suspect that an animal has rabies, or has died of it, or that a rabid animal has been on the premises during the previous eight weeks, he has power to declare those premises an "Infected Place" and to serve a notice on the occupier, the notice being served will impose severe restrictions on people and animals at the premises.

Where premises have been declared infected, the Ministry can order an animal on the premises to be detained and isolated in a secure place; no animal may be moved out or in without Ministry permission, and no animal may be killed without permission.

If permission is given to kill an animal, the head and neck must be made available for investigation if wanted. If such an animal should die naturally, the Inspector must be informed at once.

No dung from farms, pens, hurdles, etc. or kennels, baskets, rugs or collars of pets or any other substance or equipment with which the suspect or rabid animal has been in contact may be removed, without permission of the Inspector.

The premises, where the rabid or suspect rabid animal has been must be disinfected in a manner approved by the Ministry, and if the owner refuses or fails to do this work, the local authority may by law enter the premises to do the cleaning, and charge the owner the cost.

A notice must be prominently displayed declaring the premises an Infected Place, and warning of the presence, or suspected presence of rabies.

If the Inspector decides that any animal must be killed the owner must be told, but must do nothing to hinder the Inspector's purpose.

An Infected *Area* may be declared, where rabies exists, or has existed in the previous six months.

The size of the area will be decided by the Ministry and any restrictions which need to be applied to sporting and recreational facilities must be made known, and the relative information supplied to the secretary of the organisations who hold such activities.

In an infected area, the movement of animals will be controlled by order of the Minister. Dogs and cats must be kept securely within houses and kennels and not allowed contact with other animals, except those animals normally kept on the same premises.

Dogs must be muzzled when outside their own secure premises and exercised only on leads, no free running allowed at all.

If a muzzle cannot be worn, the dog cannot be exercised outside its own secure premises.

Dogs must not be taken on public vehicles unless they are muzzled; cats will only be carried in containers.

All such journeys are confined to places within the Infected Area, no farm or domestic animals may be taken outside the area as defined by the Ministry of Agriculture, Fisheries and Food, except under the authority of a license issued by a veterinary inspector.

No dog must be allowed to meet any other, except those normally kept with it.

Where dogs and cats are not controlled in the prescribed manner, the local authority, the police or the Ministry Inspector may take them into custody, where the animal will be kept for three days.

The place where such stray animals are being detained must be publicly announced and advertised, to give all owners ample opportunity to reclaim their animals within the three days allowed.

If the owner claims the animals, the local authority may require the owner to leave the dog or cat in safe custody with them for as long as is thought necessary, and the owner will have to pay for its keep and the expenses of taking the animal into custody.

If the expenses of such an animal are not paid, the local authority may destroy the animal, or dispose of it as they think fit, and the expenses will be recoverable by the local authority as a civil debt.

Animals which elude the catcher, or are too fierce to be approached may be destroyed in the best manner possible, by shooting, or by poison in a way which would not, outside of a rabies emergency, be legal.

An officer of the Ministry, or a police constable, may enter *any* private land for the purpose of catching or destroying an animal which should be taken into custody. These clauses give the power, as a last resort, to shoot stray dogs, or domestic dogs which are outside their premises and not on a lead and muzzled, and to destroy domestic or semi-wild cats in similar situations, cats being required to be on a lead if they are taken out for exercise. This destruction of 'loose' animals may take place on private or public property.

If compulsory vaccination is ordered, the owner of a dog or cat must see that it is vaccinated in a proper manner, with approved vaccine, and that any identity tag which is issued with the vaccination certificate is worn.

The Ministry has power to enter any land to seize an animal if the owner refuses to have it vaccinated, and either to arrange for the vaccination at the owner's expense, or to destroy the animal, dispose of its carcase and charge the owner for expenses incurred. Vaccination voluntarily complied with will be free to those animals which the Ministry declares should be vaccinated.

In an Infected Area, dog and cat shows, horse shows and agricultural and county shows may be banned for as long as the Ministry thinks necessary. If there is a ban, hunting, deer stalking, greyhound racing, coursing, or training for these sports, point to points, and all shooting will be stopped and anyone who takes part in any of these activities, and the owner of the land on which the event is held will be committing an offence against the law.

All animal deaths, or carcases of dead animals found within an Infected

Area, must be reported to the Ministry Inspector unless there are good grounds for knowing the animal in question did not die of rabies.

SCHEDULE 2

FORM OF NOTICE DECLARING AND DEFINING THE LIMITS OF AN INFECTED PLACE

DISEASES OF ANIMALS ACT 1950
THE RABIES (CONTROL) ORDER 1974
(Article 5)

NOTICE DECLARING AND DEFINING THE LIMITS OF AN INFECTED PLACE

To ....

of ....

....

I, the undersigned, being an inspector of the Ministry of Agriculture, Fisheries and Food (or an inspector of the local authority for the

.... of ....)
hereby give you as the occupier of the undermentioned premises notice that in accordance with the provisions of the above-mentioned order, the undermentioned premises are hereby declared to be an infected place for the purposes of the said order, *and that the premises, and any person from time to time thereat, accordingly become subject to the Rules specified in this notice which are printed on the back hereof. Any person infringing these Rules is liable to prosecution.*

This notice remains in force in its present form until it is cancelled or varied by a subsequent notice served by an inspector of the Ministry on the occupier of the infected place.

NOTE—A notice declaring an infected place may be served under Article 5 of the Rabies (Control) Order in respect of any premises at which there is an animal affected with or suspected of being affected with rabies, or at which such an animal has died, or in respect of premises at which an inspector has reasonable grounds for suspecting that rabies has existed within the previous 56 days, or that there is an animal which has been or which may have been exposed to the infection of rabies through contact with an affected or suspected animal.

Description of infected place

Dated .... 19...

(Signed) ....

Official address ....

....

NOTE—The Inspector is with all practicable speed to send copies of this notice to the Secretary, Ministry of Agriculture, Fisheries and Food, Animal Health Division, Hook Rise South, Tolworth, Surrey KT6 7NF, to the local authority, to the Divisional Veterinary Officer and to the police officer in charge of the nearest police station in the district in which the infected place is situated.

The Rules set out in Article 7 are to be printed on the back of this notice.

The Criminal Law Act which came into force in September 1977 made important new provisions both for increased fines for cruelty to animals and for those who allow dogs to worry farm stock, but also greatly increased the powers of arrest for the police in rabies cases. Maximum fines in magistrates' courts for offences against the anti-rabies legislation were increased from £400 to £1,000.

A police constable can now arrest, without need for a warrant, any person giving cause for suspicion that an offence in connection with landing an animal illegally has been or is about to be committed. The owner of a boat, or the person in charge of it, if suspected of landing an animal in Britain illegally or of moving one in or out of an infected area may be arrested on suspicion. There is also power for police to search vehicles or boats of which they are suspicious, in addition to the normal search by Customs and Excise on entry.

Now that the maximum fine for illegal entry is more than doubled to £1,000, magistrates are being urged to impose realistic fines which will greatly exceed the cost of putting an animal through quarantine, so removing part of the temptation to evade the law. The greatest deterrent of all is the certainty that the crime will be discovered and to this end the Customs and Excise force will be increasing their vigilance in ways which, for obvious reasons, they are unwilling to reveal.

Future Developments

Human rabies patients may well in future be nursed in a plastic isolator tent which was originally developed at the Royal Veterinary College for work with animals which had highly contagious disease. Calves and foals were first nursed in these tents, and with only minor adjustments, a model has now been manufactured for human use.

The tents are constructed on a plastic coated metal framework, draped in plastic sheeting, with specially constructed tunnels in the plastic through which fresh supplies may be taken in, and discarded material and samples sent out in sealed bags. The nurses who attend the patient within the isolator wear full protective clothing. A negative air pressure is maintained within the isolating plastic envelope so that no infected air can escape. When the patient has left the isolator, all the plastic covering is burnt and the framework disinfected thoroughly.

A New Treatment for Humans

It is possible that in future human rabies patients may be treated with the new drug Interferon which has proved effective in preventing the multiplication of a virus within living cells. The drug is at the moment very new and expensive; a course of treatment might well cost thousands of pounds. The hope is that a cheaper way of making Interferon may be found, using human cells by the tissue culture method, thus making Interferon available for treating virus diseases which now defeat medical science.

Vaccine for Animals

Vaccine manufacturers have been asked to have available a contingency supply of 250,000 doses of anti-rabies vaccine for animals, for emergency use should it be needed, when it could very quickly be flown from France to Britain. It is not considered necessary to store more vaccine here, for a bigger supply could be got within seven days, and it is an expensive commodity to have in bulk should it not be needed; shelf life of vaccines is not very long. Vaccine must be stored under refrigeration below 10°C, and used immediately it is reconstituted. Booster doses of vaccine will be required. In Great Britain and other countries where only inactivated vaccines are allowed, annual boosters would be necessary. Live vaccine may only require boosting every two or three years. Some brands of vaccine are put into the skin of the neck, others have to be injected into muscle, because tissue with few blood or lymph vessels, such as solid fat, can reduce the power of the vaccine, and its transmission round the body.

No vaccine can guarantee protection for every animal vaccinated, but research work is continually being carried out, giving hope for improved protection in the future.

At the moment Government policy is against vaccination of all dogs and cats in Britain at the owner's wish; veterinary surgeons are not allowed to provide this service for their clients, but this policy could be reviewed in the light of a change in our rabies-free situation. The present policy of not allowing any pre-exposure vaccination of dogs is supported by the Royal College of Veterinary Surgeons, the British Veterinary Association and the British Small Animal Veterinary Association.

Rabies Awareness

It is possible that practice runs may be organised by local authorities and MAFF on the lines of army exercises, so that paid and volunteer personnel may be aware of what will be required of them in an actual outbreak. Experience will also be gained in co-ordinating the many different facets of animal welfare and care which would be in operation in a real outbreak.

Every week that Parliament is in session, many questions are put to the Minister of Agriculture about rabies precautions. MPs will raise the subject of particular conditions applying in their own constituencies, others will question government regulations, or make suggestions for measures which might be taken. Rabies, and its possible introduction into Britain, is very much in the forefront of the minds of those who formulate our laws. Mr Gavin Strang, Parliamentary Secretary of the Ministry of Agriculture, Fisheries and Food said his department was making determined efforts to keep rabies out of the country, and to maintain our rabies free status. He believes that the country is better equipped than ever before to keep rabies out, but if the disease does get across the Channel, his Ministry was resolved to stamp it out before it takes a hold.

During the early summer of 1976, the Government launched the Rabies Awareness Campaign, even more intensive than the one mounted the year before, and in 1977 even more effort was made. The Central Office of Information produced a programme shown on TV on the Continent and elsewhere abroad, and at home, there were TV fillers to remind British holiday makers of their obligations. A high ranking officer from the rabies team of the Ministry visited his opposite number in Denmark, Holland, Belgium and France, and through that visit made contact with port authorities and Customs officials; this was a repeat visit of one which was made in 1976 and proved very effective. Concern has been expressed with regard to animals travelling in diplomatic baggage which is not, for courtesy reasons, subject to the usual customs search. There is, however, no diplomatic immunity from quarantine for animals.

Jersey (Channel Islands) dog clubs are to establish a register of experienced and willing dog owners who will be available to give practical assistance to the veterinary profession and local authority workers in the event of rabies breaking out on the island. ROVER, the Register of Organised Volunteers to Eliminate Rabies is the code word for this public spirited group in what they declare is the most rabies conscious community in the whole of Britain.

The Alsatian Training Club of Jersey has also issued thousands of car stickers with the slogan PERIL, and arranged 12 showings of the rabies films *La Rage*, and *Once Bitten*, to groups including dog clubs, schools, police and port officers, yacht clubs and the general public.

Many dog clubs throughout the UK are giving film shows and arranging for veterinary surgeons and MAFF officials to talk to them, and members of the general public are always welcome to attend. Womens Institutes and Townswomen Guilds have also mounted lecture sessions, both to give information and to dispel the many misconceptions which exist about rabies. The British Small Animal Veterinary Association has produced a tape/slide kit for veterinary audiences and will have a similar one for the general public early in 1978.

One of the practical suggestions made in Parliament was that "sniffer" dogs, trained by the police for the detection of dangerous drugs, should have their training adapted to work on locating the presence of other animals in hand luggage and in cars at the ports. Discussions are still going on with the police, but the application of dogs to this work is not as simple as it sounds. The smell of dog or cat lingers for a long time on upholstery, on rugs and even on clothing. The sniffer dog might be giving a strong indication of finding an animal which normally rode a great deal in a certain car, but had not accompanied its owners on holiday. Another point of significance is that the labradors which are normally used in this detector work must have periodic success to keep them keen. If, as we hope, people stop trying to smuggle dogs into Britain, the dogs might have to work for a long time without ever finding their quarry, and so their work would decline in vigour. When the dogs are used for drug detection, it is possible for a small quantity to be deliberately planted to keep the dogs interested, but to "plant" a smuggled animal would raise many problems. If the detector dog came into actual nose and paw contact with a smuggled animal, the dog would have to be taken out of work for at least 15 days and confined, while the dog from abroad would have to be seized and put into quarantine here. It would be examined daily and, if it was healthy after 15 days, the sniffer dog would be no longer at risk and could return to duty. The illegally imported dog could then either be re-exported, held in quarantine for six months or destroyed. Bearing in mind the enormous cost of training these very valuable sniffer dogs, it can be understood that there is some reluctance to put them at risk in this way.

The British Veterinary Association and MAFF maintain a joint Rabies Control Liaison Committee which meets regularly. Guidance notes for the veterinary profession in the event of a rabies outbreak are constantly being up-dated. The logistics of special vaccination clinics, should they ever become necessary, have been studied, so that all necessary procedures will have been worked out in advance. The BVA supported the proposal that free destruction of animals should be offered to owners who feel unable to control their animals in the way necessary under the Rabies Order. There will be no recommendation to have animals destroyed but it was thought that the offer of free destruction might deter some people turning their animals loose to add to the burden at the time of an outbreak.

The MAFF is considering offering a consultation procedure for practising veterinary surgeons who meet cases in which they do not consider there are sufficient grounds for reporting suspected rabies but, nevertheless, consider it desirable to obtain a second opinion.

Specialist advice for the horse racing industry and the greyhound racing industry is now available and similar instructions are being prepared for agriculture and nature conservancy interests.

Compensation for Destruction of Animals

In January 1977 an order was laid before Parliament setting out the rates of compensation for animals which are slaughtered by order of Ministry officials during a rabies outbreak, the object of such slaughter being to prevent spread of the disease by known infected animals, or very close contacts. There will be no mass slaughter of owned and well cared for pets which have not been in contact with rabies suspects, or have not run free in an area where rabid animals are known to be loose.

The order applies to farm livestock and horses as well as pet dogs and cats. If the animal definitely has rabies, compensation will be paid at half the market value immediately before rabies was contracted. This is a generous settlement, as the animal would die anyway.

If the animal is not rabid, but must be destroyed as a close contact, full market value at the time will be paid. Compensation is only applicable to those animals ordered to be killed by the Ministry, *not* any animal killed at its owner's wish because they are worried about rabies, nor for unclaimed stray animals.

No compensation will be paid for animals smuggled in illegally, or those subject to quarantine.

Chapter 12

What Other Countries Are Doing

A World Health Organisation consultation took place in West Germany in the Autumn of 1976 to establish a data bank on European rabies. Denmark, Holland, Luxembourg, France, Austria, Poland, Czechoslovakia, Switzerland and West Germany will participate in a one year's trial which will record cases in man and animals, publish regular reports on the current situation, and evaluate the effectiveness of protective measures and establish an emergency rabies service.

In Holland, all dogs are being vaccinated against rabies under an order which came into force in May 1976.

West Germany allows the vaccination of all susceptible animals, not only dogs and cats, with inactivated rabies vaccine, dogs and cats only may be immunized with live vaccine. Animals that are suspected of having rabies must either be killed at once, or put into quarantine for three months, whether vaccinated or not. Public dog and cat shows are permitted provided the authorities are notified eight weeks in advance and the district is free from rabies.

France allows vaccination of all animals at the owner's wish. There is a very large, concentrated drive to rid France of stray dogs and cats, allowing only a 48 hour stay of execution between straying animals being picked up and euthanasia being given to unwanted animals.

In Spain, rabies vaccination is compulsory, and must be renewed every year, and, in large towns, no dogs are allowed to be exercised off the lead.

America has rabies and is never likely to be free of the disease, which reaches peaks and then subsides for a time. Rabid skunks on the fringe of a city attack cattle, horses and domestic animals, which then bite people. In the opinion of the veterinary profession, the disease is only kept within manageable limits by the willingness of owners who live in well-to-do suburbs to have their dogs vaccinated, so providing a living healthy barrier between the farm stock and the inner core of lower class housing where the percentage of vaccinated dogs and general good pet care is low. Some states in U.S.A. require evidence of anti-rabies vaccination before a dog's licence can be renewed, so it is the responsible owner, with the licensed and protected pet, who keeps rabies at bay.

In the city of Houston, Texas, 70 local authority employees are retained on rabies suppression work, 40 of them being dog wardens, engaged on rounding up 40,000 strays in 1975, and vaccinating 10,000 dogs and cats, and giving euthanasia to the 35,000 unclaimed in the course of one year. The annual budget to the city for this work was $900,000 in 1975, a considerable charge on community funds.

In an outbreak of rabies on the Texas-Mexico border in 1974, cases of rabies were encountered along 80 miles of the border and, in El Paso City, 234 dogs, six cats, 13 bats, three goats, one cow, one horse and two skunks were positively identified as rabid by laboratory tests. More than 300 humans received treatment for exposure to rabies, out of a total of 15,000 people bitten who had to be screened and examined to see if treatment was necessary. Most of the rabid dogs were young, under a year old, and quite a lot of people were bitten by pups of less than three months old, at the time puppies are play-nibbling, and not biting in any ferocious sense. Most of the rabid dogs were owned, and not strays, but few had been vaccinated against rabies, although pups can be protected, if necessary, as young as eight weeks old. The spread of rabies began by just one case being found, then several weeks later another three, then nine or 10, and then reports of cases came snowballing in. Sometimes the spread of cases can be checked by a vaccinated dog resisting the infection even though it has been bitten by a rabid animal. Several such dogs can cause a significant barrier to the spread of the disease. In America informed opinion states that vaccination and control of strays are the basic keys to control of rabies, neither succeeding without the other.

Bibliography

Aoki, F. Y. and Gamet, A. D. M., "Rabies in Man," *The Nursing Times*, 13 May 1976.

Bahmanyar, M., "Measures Against Rabies," *British Journal of Hospital Medicine*, September 1970.

Bedford, Dr. P. G. C., FRCVS, "Diagnosis of Rabies in Animals," *Veterinary Record*, August 1976.

Blackie, Dr Marjorie, *The Patient, Not the Cure*, Macdonald and Janes, 1977.

Brooks, Stewart, *The World of Viruses*, A. S. Barnes, 1970.

Caras, Roger, *Dangerous to Man*, Barrie & Jenkins, rev. ed. 1976.

Clater, Francis, *Every Man His Own Farrier*.

Hillaby, John, *Journey Through Love*, Constable, 1976.

Ladies Kennel Journal, vols. 1-4, 1894-96.

Leach, Maria, *God Had a Dog*, Rutgers University Press.

Minor, R., MA VetMB MRCVS, "Clinical Rabies of Possible Vaccinal Origin in Two Dogs," letter to *Veterinary Record*, 28 August 1976.

———, "Rabies in the Dog," *Veterinary Record*, vol. 101, 1977.

Parish, H. J., *A History of Immunisation*, Churchill Livingstone, 1967.

Proceedings of the Royal Society of Health Symposium on Rabies, 1976.

Rabies Control and Greyhound Racing, National Greyhound Racing Club Ltd.

Report of the BSAVA Rabies Working Party, 1976.

Rhodes, A. J. and Van Rooyen, C. E., *Textbook of Virology*, The Williams Wilkins Co.

Sigerist, Henry, *The Great Doctors*, Dover Publications.

Stockman, M. J. R., MRCVS, "Visit to Institute Merrieux," *Veterinary Drug*, July 1976.

Swain, R. H. A., *Clinical Virology*, Churchill Livingstone, 1967.

Taylor, G., MRCVS, "Rabies, the Epizootic Aspects," *Veterinary Record*, 28 August 1976.

Turner, G. S., Aoki, F. *et al.*, "Human Diploid Cell Vaccine," *The Lancet*, 26 June 1976.

The Veterinary Contribution to Public Health, World Health Organisation, 1975.

West, Geoffrey P., *Rabies in Animals and Man*, David & Charles, 1972.

Williams, Veronica Tudor, *Basenjis*, David & Charles.

Youatt, William, *The Dog*, 1854.